ANATOMY
— of a —
JOB SEARCH

ANATOMY
—of a—
JOB SEARCH

*A Nurse's Guide to Finding and
Landing the Job You Want*

JEANNA BOZELL, RN, CPC

*President, Professional Resource Group, Inc.
President, Indiana Association of Personnel Services*

SPRINGHOUSE CORPORATION Springhouse, Pennsylvania

STAFF

Vice President
Matthew Cahill

Editorial Director
Darlene Cooke

Clinical Director
Judith Schilling McCann, RN, MSN

Art Director
John Hubbard

Managing Editor
David Moreau

Acquisitions Editor
Patricia Kardish Fischer, RN, BSN

Editor
Margaret MacKay Eckman

Copy Editors
Brenna H. Mayer (manager),
Stacy A. Follin, Barbara Long,
Kathy Marino, Pamela Wingrod

Designers
Arlene Putterman (associate art
director), Debra Moloshok (designer),
Susan Hopkins Rodzewich (project
manager), Donna S. Morris

Manufacturing
Deborah Meiris (director),
Patricia K. Dorshaw (manager),
Otto Mezei (book production manager)

Editorial Assistants
Beverly Lane, Marcia Mills,
Liz Schaeffer

The procedures described and recommended in this publication are based on research and consultation with nursing authorities. To the best of our knowledge, these procedures reflect currently accepted practice; nevertheless, they cannot be considered absolute and universal recommendations. The author and the publisher disclaim responsibility for adverse effects resulting directly or indirectly from the suggested procedures, from any undetected errors, or from the reader's misunderstanding of the text.

Printed in the United States of America.

AJS-010399

A member of the Reed Elsevier plc group

Library of Congress Cataloging-in-Publication Data

Bozell, Jeanna.
  Anatomy of a job search: a nurse's guide to finding and
  landing the job you want/ Jeanna Bozell.
    p.   cm.
  Includes index.
  1. Nursing—Vocational guidance. 2. Nurses—Employment.
  3. Job hunting.
  [DNLM: 1. Job Application nurses' instruction.WY29 B793a 1999]
RT86.7.B69 1999
610.73'06'9-dc21
DNLM/DLC   98-48422
ISBN 0-87434-950-8 (alk. paper)   CIP

CONTENTS

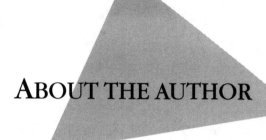

ABOUT THE AUTHOR

Jeanna Bozell, RN, CPC, a nurse recruiter since 1989, is a certified personnel consultant through the National Association of Personnel Services, achieving the highest standard of the recruitment industry. As an RN, she experienced the clinical arena before becoming a placement consultant. She is president and founder of Professional Resource Group, Inc., a search firm specializing in the national placement of candidates in nursing management and advanced practice nursing. Jeanna currently serves as president of the Indiana Association of Personnel Services.

Professional Resource Group, Inc., is proud to be a member of the National Association of Personnel Services, the Indiana Association of Personnel Services, the Indiana Chamber of Commerce, and the Muncie-Delaware County Chamber of Commerce.

For further information, contact:

> *Jeanna Bozell, RN, CPC*
> Professional Resource Group, Inc.
> P.O. Box 1007
> Muncie, IN 47308-1007
> Phone: (800) 776-0127
> E-mail: jbozell@nursequest.com

To the One who taught me love,

patience, kindness, compassion, and forgiveness.

You really are the way, the truth, and the life.

With you in my heart, I am forever changed.

❖

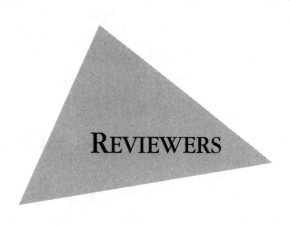

REVIEWERS

Dawna Martich, RN, MSN
Clinical Manager
University of Pittsburgh Medical Center
University Family Practice Associates, Inc.

Nila Saliba
Healthcare Recruitment Manager
University of Virginia Medical Center
Charlottesville

ACKNOWLEDGMENTS

My deepest appreciation:

- to the nurses and employers whom I have had the honor and privilege of getting to know. Together we have learned from your trials and tribulations and your successes.
- to my own nursing instructors, especially Mary Jane Knapp.
- to my trusted colleagues and mentors in the search industry.
- to the participants of the Midwest Writers' Workshop, especially Holly Miller, Dennis Hensley, and Brenda Poinsett, who unselfishly share their knowledge with new writers.
- to Pat Wendleken, my friend and confidant, for her wisdom and support during this undertaking.
- to Trish Fischer, my acquisitions editor, for her patience, encouragement, and belief in this project.
- to my office staff: Tammy Resler, Tina Farmer, and Robin Baker.
- to the memory of my father for all he taught me about life and business; to my mother for showing me perseverance and a positive attitude, no matter what the circumstances.
- to the joys of my life, my children — Robin, Brandon, and Shawnee — and my grandchildren — Whitney, Jordan, Bren, and Mariah.
- and especially to Jerry, my husband and best friend, for serving as my "in-house" Human Resources Director, my editor, and my most honest critic. His love and encouragement have enabled yet another of my dreams to come true.

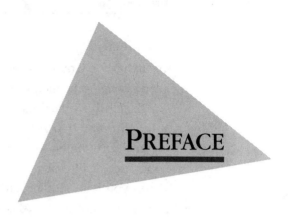

PREFACE

As an RN and a national nurse recruiter, I recognize the lack of job-hunting resources designed specifically for nurses. Candidates must obtain bits and pieces of often-conflicting information from one source or another. Nursing educators tell me they lack the information they need to fully prepare their students to enter the job market.

Why is this the case? First, because only a short time ago nurses didn't need résumés at all, so no format for the nursing résumé existed. The main model for a résumé is geared to business positions. But nursing is different. Employers need more detailed, descriptive information about a nurse's background to determine if the candidate meets their specific needs. Second, nurses don't fit the basic rule most employers use for hiring a candidate — the 60:40 rule. When I first entered the recruiting arena, I was told that if a candidate is 60% of what the employer is looking for, I should submit that candidate. But as an RN, I know that nurses deal with life and death. A health care employer won't settle for a warm body to fill a position; nurses face more stringent hiring guidelines. The 60:40 rule doesn't apply.

So as a nurse, you're left to patch together your job search without the right tools. You're faced with literally hundreds of generic career "how-to" books on the market to weed through, looking for one on résumé preparation, another on job-hunting, a third on writing a cover letter, and still another book on interviewing—and then you have to adapt their advice to nursing. Exactly how much time do you have to invest?

In *Anatomy of a Job Search: A Nurse's Guide to Finding and Landing the Job You Want,* I hope to change that. A book specifically for nurses, *Anatomy of a Job Search* furnishes you with all the pertinent information you need for your search—one-stop shopping, so to speak.

Chapter 1 covers a few preliminaries. How's the nursing market? What can a student do while still in school to better her chances of securing a job? What do you need to know if you want to transition to another clinical area? What do you need to know if you were downsized or reorganized out of your position? How do you proactively manage the stress of a job change?

Chapter 2 leads you through a professional and personal assessment of your current situation. Do you really want to make a change? Should you? What do you need to think about before you decide?

Chapter 3 guides you step by step through developing your résumé and cover letters, including samples of each, and advises you on choosing your references.

Chapter 4 helps you plan for your search, covering networking options, responding to advertisements, using the Internet, and choosing professional recruiters.

Chapter 5 shows you how to prepare for the telephone and on-site interviews.

Chapter 6 deals with negotiating the best offer, leaving your current employer (including a sample letter of resignation), and planning for the future.

 IN REAL LIFE   Throughout the book, you'll see the *In real life* logo beside examples of actual candidate experiences (the names and a few of the details have been changed to maintain confidentiality). These examples can help you learn from others' mistakes — a lot less painful than learning from your own.

INSIDE TRACK The *Inside track* logo highlights helpful job search tips. These proven job winners will give you an extra advantage during your job search, putting you on the inside track to landing the job you want.

FIRST TIMER Students, a *First timer* logo within the text marks areas geared especially to your needs, although each chapter contains valuable information for all nurses.

ON THE MOVE If you're thinking about relocating, look for the *On the move* logo. It appears in the text beside information specifically related to relocating.

I've written *Anatomy of a Job Search* in a conversational style to match the way I talk with my candidates, from the Student Nurse to the Vice President of Nursing. Also, because most health care hiring officials and nurses are women, I've generally used the feminine pronoun.

I've done my best to pass on to you what I've learned from both employers and candidates — a behind-the-scenes look at what they liked, what they didn't like, and what they wish they could have done differently. What better way to learn what works in a nursing job search than from this unique perspective?

I hope you can use this book as a resource now and throughout your career. Writing this book for you has truly been a privilege, and I wish you the best in all of your searches!

Jeanna Bozell, RN, CPC

1
THE PRELIMINARIES

Nancy Ramsey had been a nurse for almost 9 years. After 5 years at the same hospital, she felt it was time for a change. A friend told her about an interesting position in a nearby hospital, one she thought she could handle with a little training. So she called the hospital and arranged for an interview. Nancy arrived on time, relaxed and confident, no résumé in hand—and got the job.

At least, that's how it used to work. But nursing has changed and grown. Nurses need to know more than ever as medicine evolves. Many specialties, such as Nurse Practitioner, offer nurses increased autonomy and responsibility. Along with the increased responsibility, salaries have also risen. Nursing has evolved into a valued and respected profession—and more and more graduates, armed with bachelor's, master's, even doctoral degrees, are entering the profession.

To get the position you want in today's competitive job market, your professionalism must show in your educational background, job history, performance, and presentation. You need to have the skills and background the employer wants, with a résumé to prove it. In short, you must be prepared.

As part of that preparation, take the time to go over these preliminary questions before diving into the assessment and job search techniques covered in the following chapters.

- How is the nursing job market changing? What clinical areas are in demand? What areas will be in demand in the future?

 FIRST TIMER If you're a student, you have no work experience and no employment references. What can you do before you graduate to improve your chances? ❖

- Are you considering a switch to another clinical area, whether by choice or necessity? How can you prepare yourself to increase your marketability?

- Have you been downsized or reorganized out of a job? What steps should you take before looking for a new position?

- How will you deal with the stress of the job search? The emotional impact of leaving your old job, even your home if you relocate? The effect on your family? Thinking about these questions beforehand can help you to be proactive instead of reactive.

As you can see, some questions are geared to specific situations — the student preparing to enter the workforce for the first time, for instance.

But all of these questions can give you insight into what's happening in the nursing profession today and can help prepare you for your search.

A CHANGING MARKET

A decade ago, Nurse Practitioners were in little demand, and few candidates pursued careers in that specialty. Staff Nurses, Nurse Managers, and Nurse Administrators were in short supply, and the need for the Clinical Nurse Specialist began to grow.

But the nursing market changed. The demand for Nurse Practitioners escalated as managed care organizations and independent medical practices learned about the advantages of the position. In response, Nurse Practitioner programs multiplied rapidly, supplying the market with enough candidates to meet that need. Mergers, downsizing, and restructuring reduced the number of openings for Nurse Administrators. Financial cutbacks also decreased the demand for Clinical Nurse Specialists as positions were eliminated or left unfilled. Many employers began to demand a minimum of 1 year of clinical background in such specialties as critical care, emergency department nursing, and obstetrics, making it more difficult for nurses just receiving their RN licenses to get jobs.

And all this will change — again.

Emerging needs

Of course, some geographic areas are near saturation, with few nursing jobs available. But overall, nurses are in short supply, and that shortage will grow. (See *Where should I look?* page 4.)

The demand for Staff Nurses in particular will increase more than ever before. Why? Several factors come into play: The baby boomers outnumber the next generation almost three to one, and the current unemployment rate remains low. As baby boomers age and retire, they leave behind many more positions than there are workers in the following generation to fill those positions. Plus, these newly retired boomers face all the health problems of aging. So, the number of workers decreases at the same time the patient population grows, leading to a huge demand for health care workers. Talk about job security!

Demand for the Clinical Nurse Specialist is also increasing. Not only is she a resource person in a specific clinical area, the Clinical Nurse Specialist also develops and maintains nurse practice standards and performs research and case management — vital functions in nursing. The administrative market, on the other hand, is in flux. The Nurse Manager po-

WHERE SHOULD I LOOK?

Where will the best nursing jobs be in the future? The following areas hold the promise of growth:
- Ambulatory care
- Ambulatory surgery
- Case management
- Critical care nursing
- Geriatric care, skilled nursing care, and long-term care
- Home health care
- Obstetrics
- Operating room nursing
- Quality improvement
- Rehabilitation
- Subacute care.

sition is holding its own in the marketplace, but many of the Vice Presidents and Directors of Nursing forced out because of mergers and downsizing are getting out of the hospital setting, returning to school, or becoming consultants. Recognizing the trends is your best bet for finding the right job in an ever-changing market.

GETTING THAT FIRST JOB

As a student, you face particular challenges. You've probably never had to prepare a nursing résumé and may not know where to start. You haven't been through the interview process. And, perhaps most challenging of all, you have little or no work experience.

Chapter 3, The Tools, will help you develop your résumé, and chapter 5, The Interviews, will discuss interview recommendations and practical insights. But you can take steps now, as a student, to overcome that lack of work experience. Careful planning can help you obtain the right first job.

References

One of the first steps you can take is to get the best references you can. With little or no work experience, your references become one of the main sources a potential employer has to decide whether to hire you. So you must gather strong professional references—not from friends or relatives but from your instructors, who know your work.

Think carefully about which instructors to ask for references. You should have a sense of how your instructors will answer the questions a potential employer might ask. (See *What will my instructor say?*)

If you don't like the answers you think your instructors might give, then you may need to reassess yourself as a student. Juggling classes, doing clinical rotations, and perhaps working a part-time job can be exhausting; you may have skipped a class here and there to catch up on commitments, or you just may have overslept. But with little or no work experience, references from your instructors play a crucial

IN REAL LIFE

WHAT WILL MY INSTRUCTOR SAY?

Potential employers want to know if you would make a good employee, and they will ask some tough questions to find out. Think about how your instructors may answer the following:
- Is she dependable? Does she attend classes regularly? How often is she absent? Does she get to class and clinical rotations on time?
- How does she get along with peers? With patients and their families? With you and her other instructors?
- What are her strengths?
- Does she have weaknesses that could affect her job performance?
- Does she present a professional image?
- Would you hire her?

role in convincing a potential employer to hire you; they must be excellent, and you must be the best student you can be to get those references. (See the section on letters of reference in chapter 3, The Tools.)

Clinical experience

Another way to help make up for your lack of full-time work experience is to get as much clinical experience as possible. If you can secure a part-time job as a Student Nurse Extern, all the better: You'll gain some actual work experience while you're still in school. If you're already an LPN in an RN program, you might want to continue working as an LPN.

The right experience

Getting some work experience can help enormously, but make sure it's moving you forward in your career path. For example, if you want to become a Pediatric Nurse Practitioner, don't work part-time in a nursing home. Yes, it's experience, but it might as well be in auto racing! If you want to become a Pediatric Nurse Practitioner, try to find part-time work, even volunteer work, in pediatrics.

Working in the specialty in which you're interested also gives you a chance to find the right mentor, one who already works in that specialty. A good mentor can give you a wealth of knowledge. Explain your goals and ask for her help. You'll probably find that she'll bend over backward to assist you. And once you've learned from her and she's learned about you and your abilities, you can ask for a letter of recommendation to submit with your résumé. Work experience in the specialty you're interested in, help from the right mentor, and a good letter of recommendation from that mentor can all weigh heavily in your favor, maybe enough to tip the scale in your direction and get you the job you're looking for.

Clinical rotations

A final thought on how you can prepare as a student for your job search: Your clinical rotations, some of which you may have chosen yourself, can gain you not only experience but also an excellent chance for employment. The staff—and maybe the person who does the hiring—can get to know you and your abilities. So work hard during your clinical rotations. You may find your first job right there.

TRANSITIONS

Changes in health care are causing nurses at all levels to find themselves in transition from one clinical area to another. Whether such a transition is by choice or necessity, it can mean major changes in your professional life. Before you decide to switch to a different clinical area, you may want to think about how feasible such a change would be and how it would affect you. Read further to learn more about the unique characteristics of home care, long-term care, and critical care, and learn how you can make the transition from the more traditional acute care and medical-surgical care settings to these growing areas.

From acute care to home health care

As the need for home health care grows, many nurses are choosing to move from the hospital setting to home health care. Before you decide if you want to switch, take a look at what it's like to work in home health care:

- Patients tend to be older. If you don't like working with older patients, don't consider this area.
- Patients come from many different cultural backgrounds. As a guest in their homes, you must show respect for their beliefs and their cultures.

- You need dependable transportation and must drive in all kinds of weather at any time, day or night.
- You should have excellent assessment skills and know when something isn't right. You must have confidence in your decisions — no one's around to validate your conclusions — and be able to work independently with fewer resources.
- You must feel comfortable working alone.
- You must take responsibility for your safety and the safety of your equipment. If you have to work in dangerous neighborhoods, you must always be aware of your surroundings.
- You must assess the patient's environment for unsafe conditions, just as you would a hospital room. You may find it harder to pinpoint and control hazards in the patient's home than in a hospital because the home is a less controlled environment.
- Get ready for lots of paperwork; to be reimbursed, you must create thorough plans of care and document everything.
- Patients and home caregivers have to care for I.V. lines, catheters, and other equipment, increasing the risk of infection; you'll need to take extra precautions to help prevent or control infection.
- You'll need to adjust to a slower pace than you may be used to; patient care is more relaxed at home than in the hospital.

Who is the best candidate for home health care?

An ideal background for moving into home health care is an RN license, plus a minimum of 4 years of clinical experience in medical-surgical or critical care nursing. Excellent I.V. skills and experience with central venous lines, total parenteral nutrition, and chemotherapy is preferred. A good candidate should also have strong patient education skills to teach patients to perform some of their own home care. Important personal attributes include confidence, independent thinking, problem-solving skills, common sense, compassion, and flexibility. Finally, a good home health care nurse should know when it's necessary to call the doctor.

If you have the right personal attributes and want to work in home health care, get the certifications and experience you need. When you draft your résumé, list all appropriate certifications, such as "certified in medical-surgical nursing," and name each skill you've acquired, such as "served on I.V. team for emergency services" and "performed patient education." The potential employer will scan incoming résumés for these specific experiences.

This doesn't mean you won't be hired if you lack some of these skills. But it does mean that someone with more of these skills stands a better chance than you do. Particularly in home health care, employers prefer candidates with experience because they must work in the field with minimal support.

If you want to work in home health care administration but only have administrative experience in acute care, you face more of a challenge. Unless you know someone who can help get you up and running, you may have a difficult time finding a position because essentially you're applying for a job for which you have little experience. So you'll probably have to start at the staff level and work your way up, even if you're currently a Director of Nursing at a hospital. On the plus side, once you've learned the basics of home health care, you already have the administrative background to move easily into that administrative position.

 FIRST TIMER If you're a student, you can help prepare yourself by applying for a clinical rotation in home health.

Don't wait for the opportunities to come to you—go looking for them. ❖

From acute care to long-term care

With a growing elderly population and a shortage of nurses working in long-term care, you have an excellent opportunity to switch! Look over what it's like to work in long-term care to help you decide if you want to work in this specialty.

- As in home health care, long-term care patients tend to be elderly. Consider this area only if you like working with older patients.
- You'll have a much heavier patient load than you would in a hospital.
- As in home health care, you must document meticulously.
- As the name implies, patients stay for a long time, unlike in a typical hospital setting.

Some facilities also have subacute units. If you want to work with a more acute and diverse patient population, you may want to consider this as an alternative to working on a long-term care unit.

Who is the best candidate for long-term care?

A good candidate should have a solid medical-surgical clinical background; charge nurse experience or supervisory experience is another plus. If you have some of these other skills and characteristics, long-term care might be a good match for you. (See *Switching to long-term care.*)

 FIRST TIMER   Students, this area is yours for the choosing—and the opportunities will only improve as baby boomers age. Get some experience while still in school by working as a Nursing Assistant or a Student Nurse at a long-term care facility; they're almost always looking for caring, high-quality professionals. Learn all you can while you're there. ❖

IN REAL LIFE

SWITCHING TO LONG-TERM CARE

Thinking of a switch to long-term care? Check this list for some of the skills and personal characteristics that can help you succeed.

Skills
- Assessment
- I.V. care
- Care planning
- Computer

Personal characteristics
- Organized
- Prioritizes well
- Flexible
- Not easily overwhelmed
- Works well with others
- Pitches in where needed

From medical-surgical to critical care

Switching from medical-surgical nursing to critical care is not quite as drastic as moving from acute care to home health care or long-term care, but you'll still need to consider the differences in working in critical care.

- You'll be caring for critically ill patients, which can be very stressful.
- Conflict resolution is an important aspect of the job.
- You'll have fewer patients, but they'll need much more intensive care.
- Because these patients are acutely ill, you'll see more of them die than you would in other nursing areas because they are acutely ill. Think about how well you handle death and how you would be at comforting dying patients and their families.
- You may have to face the ethical dilemma of whether or not to remove life-support systems.
- Work is fast-paced and intense, and you'll need to make many nursing decisions quickly.

- The ever-changing environment requires great flexibility; a patient can go from stable condition to critical condition in a heartbeat.

Who is the best candidate for critical care?

To work in critical care, you should have a strong medical-surgical clinical background with excellent assessment and I.V. skills. Taking a class in basic electrocardiography and earning your certification in advanced cardiac life support can help. You can also prepare by working on a progressive or step-down unit, where patients are more acutely ill than medical-surgical patients but not as gravely ill as critical care patients. Such work can help accustom you to more acutely ill patients as well as the monitors and medications used in critical care.

Critical care work isn't for everyone. You have to be a self-starter with a good work ethic, work well under stress, and be a proactive, critical thinker who asks questions when necessary.

 FIRST TIMER   Students, if you want to work in critical care, try working as a Student Nurse on a progressive care unit or a critical care unit for a weekend or two a month. You'll learn a lot of the basics and will work more closely with critical care nurses and doctors. ❖

Coping with unemployment

Losing a job can be devastating, especially when you know it wasn't your fault. Many of us were brought up to believe that in a layoff situation, if you were a good employee, the employer would find a position for you. Today, you're laid off and on your own.

How you handle yourself throughout this process will affect your search. You can't control what the employer may do, but you *can* choose how to react. First, gather as many reference letters as possible—from peers, supervisors, sub-ordinates, and doctors—as soon as you receive notice of your termination. Don't wait until after you've left; absence doesn't always make the heart grow fonder.

The right attitude

Next, recognize the rush of emotions a job loss brings—shock, hurt, sadness, then bitterness and anger—and take the time to work through those feelings before you begin a new job search so that you can go forward with the right attitude. If you go into the interview with a chip on your shoulder, all the hiring official will see is an angry candidate with a bad attitude. She doesn't know what's going on to cause those feelings. Some candidates in these circumstances have even demanded proof from the interviewer that the job would be guaranteed for years if they took the position. But no employer can make a guarantee like that.

When you've worked through your feelings—however long it takes—write down how you'll explain the situation, truthfully and objectively, without seeming negative. Start with one sentence about why you're not working, and mention two or three things you learned while you were employed at your previous position. Don't overexplain or you'll sound like you're covering something up. Then, read it aloud, listening to the tone of your voice. Even if what you've written is terrific, an angry and bitter tone will give you away. You don't have to be happy about what happened, but if you're comfortable with it, you can give a good response when the hiring official asks why you're not employed. (See *How you come across,* page 14.) You may even find out that, in the long run, losing your job was one of the best things that ever happened to you.

How you come across

When you're asked to explain why you left your old position, what you say — and how you say it — can make all the difference. See how the difference in attitude comes across in these two examples.

Poor response
"I worked there for 6 years. We merged with the other hospital in town, and they fired our whole team without warning. There's just no loyalty. I put in 60 hours a week, and look where it got me."

Good response
"We merged with another facility in town that had a more senior management team. But I learned a great deal in the past 6 years and was fortunate enough to be involved in many special projects. Our team developed a case management program, and I was involved in the startup of our new ambulatory surgery center. All things considered, it was a very positive experience."

MANAGING STRESS

Changing jobs ranks high on the scale of stressful life events, up near getting a divorce or the death of a family member. The stresses related to a job change can even interfere with your ability to make decisions. If you don't think through what kinds of situations you might face *before* they happen, you may find yourself making a bad decision — like turning down a wonderful position because you're feeling too stressed to face the change.

Your family's reaction

How you manage the stress of a job change is one thing. But how will your family react, and how will you handle that reaction? If you're really going to change jobs, you must have the support of your family, especially your spouse. Take the time to ensure that your family is with you 100%, or you'll all face more problems down the road.

ON THE MOVE   If a job change means relocating and you have children, especially teenagers in high school, you face more decisions — and added stress. You may choose not to relocate until after school ends. Or you may decide to leave your spouse and children behind for a few months and have them join you right after school lets out for the summer. If you do this, keep in mind that the summer can seem pretty long to a child who's new in town. If you move before the school year ends, your children may have a chance to make some friends at school to play with during the summer. ❖

If you live close to your parents or in-laws, how will they react to the news that you're moving? Picture yourself telling them that you've just received a great job offer—in another state. Some planning on your part will make the process easier for the entire family. (See *Don't leave us!* page 16.)

Expect the unexpected

Keep in mind that, no matter how much you plan—and planning really can help you deal with some of the stresses of changing jobs—you can't foresee everything. In fact, some of the most unexpected reactions may be your own. You'll need to be flexible and creative. One candidate found herself in a dilemma when she got a job offer in another state that she really wanted to accept, but she couldn't bear the thought of leaving her house. The solution? She built the exact same house at her new destination—with a few modifications to make it even better. Talk about feeling "at home" in a new community!

If you have to relocate, you may find ending close relationships within your community more painful than you imag-

DON'T LEAVE US!

If you receive a job offer that requires you to relocate away from your children's grandparents, don't be surprised if they don't react quite the way you did to your news. You may actually say something like, "I have a great job offer in another state! It's the next logical step in my career, and I'll get a good salary increase, more responsibility, autonomy, and wonderful growth potential. It's just what I've worked so hard for. We're so excited!" But all they may hear is "We're taking your grandchildren away from you, and you'll never see or hear from them again."

You'll need to help them cope with their feelings of abandonment. One way is to have a plan for family visits ready *before* you break the news, which can help reassure them that they won't lose you. Tell them about the things they'd like in your new town — maybe it's near a retirement resort that has lots of activities they'd love. Be creative; add any positives. Try to put yourself in their shoes and think about how they'll react to your news. If you aren't prepared for their reaction, you'll find it difficult — if not impossible — to come up with an immediate response.

ined. It's important to recognize these feelings and let yourself say goodbye. But then you need to move forward and see the move as a chance for a new beginning, the chance to build new relationships.

Whether or not you relocate, a job change means leaving your boss and coworkers, who have been through a lot with you — some good, some bad. If the job change is your choice, how will you feel when you tell your boss you're leaving, especially if your boss is a good friend? How might your boss react? With anger? Support?

The actual moment of resignation can cause a lot of stress. (You'll find more about resignations in chapter 6, The Offer [and Beyond].) Think through it before it happens — what

WHAT A SHOCK

A Trauma Nurse Coordinator for 8 years, Chris had no opportunity for advancement, so he looked for a position that would allow him to advance in his career. After finding a promising position, he tendered a month's notice, as hospital policy required. His supervisor accepted his resignation — and then politely told him to pack his things and leave at once.

Shocked, Chris spoke with the Director of Human Resources. He told her what high evaluations he had received, reminded her of his spotless attendance record, and explained that he had given appropriate notice. Despite all this, he was again told to leave immediately.

The hospital paid Chris for the month's notice, but he hadn't been ready for the hospital to let him go like that. He took it as a personal insult and left the job with many of his fond memories of the hospital soured by the experience.

you'll say and what your employer might say in response. Don't take anything personally, and don't let any reaction catch you off guard. (See *What a shock.*)

Throughout the process, the strength of your emotional reactions may surprise you. So expect the unexpected, even in yourself, and try to recognize and deal with your emotions so that you can discern between emotional pulls and professional goals. If you're not ready for some of these emotional "sneak attacks," they may interfere with your ability to make realistic and objective decisions. If you can't bring yourself to make the break, find out now. Every situation is unique; you need to do what's best for you.

A day at a time

Of course, you should prepare as much as possible and be flexible enough to deal with unexpected twists and turns. Preparing helps prevent you from getting all the way to the offer stage before realizing the seriousness of the situation and only then thinking of everything involved. Preparing helps you deal with leaving your current job and the relationships you've built with your boss and coworkers, with possibly selling your house, with finding a new place to live, and with starting your children in a new school. But you should also let yourself take it one day at a time, or you may be completely overwhelmed, despite the best preparation.

Do you remember how overwhelmed you felt sitting in class on the first day of college? You looked over the syllabus the professor handed out: Read your text plus two additional books, write three reports, and take two tests plus a final. And that was just for one class! But you did it. And you can handle the stress of a job change the same way: You need to plan—but take it one day at a time.

2

THE ASSESSMENTS

Before you begin your job search, you need to assess your situation—both professionally and personally. You need to know what you're looking for in order to find it. Such an assessment helps you to focus on what's important to you.

This chapter guides you step-by-step through the assessment process. The professional assessment lets you pinpoint what you need in a position—what would make a potential position ideal and what would detract from it, maybe enough for you to turn the job down. If a new job would require you to relocate, then the assessment becomes more personal. You need to decide if you and your family are willing to uproot and start again in a new location.

This detailed assessment process can help you develop your personal "blueprint" that can guide you throughout the search and keep you focused on what you really want. Without it, you may find yourself expending tremendous effort on your job search before you've answered the most basic questions. You may be faced with deciding whether to accept a job—or even deciding between two job offers — and not know what to do. Without a blueprint, you may be tempted, for instance, to compare two job offers and accept the better of the two when you should be measuring *both* jobs against your blueprint. By comparing both jobs with what you really want, you may even find that neither position mea-

I CAN WAIT

Steve was just starting a search for his first Family Nurse Practitioner position. He knew that Nurse Practitioners were in demand and received an excellent job offer after his first on-site interview. The position offered Steve most of what he was looking for in a job. But he didn't measure the job against his blueprint. Instead, he turned the offer down without seriously considering it. "After all," he rationalized, "It's only the first position I've looked at. If I found a good position that quickly, something even better is bound to be out there. I can wait."

A full year and many interviews later, he took a position that didn't meet his criteria nearly as well as that first position. But by then, he needed to take a job.

sures up, and you'll have saved yourself from making a bad decision. Take a look at what can happen if you lose sight of what you really want. (See *I can wait.*)

PROFESSIONAL ASSESSMENT

The professional assessment will help you pinpoint your goals and discover what will motivate you to accept a new position or keep you in your current situation. Key questions can help you decide why you're searching for a new job—including whether you really should be searching for a new job at all—and what kind of job you really want. As you answer these questions, remember your goal—not just to find any job but to find an exciting new opportunity. You owe it to yourself to select carefully.

Why are you in the job market?

This most basic question, along with the following specific questions, helps you understand why you're looking and what would motivate you to take a position.

FIRST TIMER   Are you a new graduate looking for your first "real" job? While you think about this question, ask yourself where you want to be in 5 years and what you need to do now, in this first job, to get there. ❖

- Do you want to return to the workforce after being unemployed for an extended time?
- Have you been "downsized" or suspect that you may be?
- Has your spouse been transferred or taken a new position?
- Are you looking for more responsibility? If you are, what kind of responsibilities would pose an exciting challenge, and what kind would overwhelm you? Be realistic about yourself and look for a position that would be a next logical step in your career—not a leap of faith. For instance, if you have never been a Manager before, it wouldn't make sense to apply for a Director of Nursing position in a 100-bed community hospital.
- Are you feeling restless or unhappy in your current position? If so, think carefully about why. You need to understand what's causing the problem before you can determine the best solution. If you don't take the time to think about it now, you may end up with a new job that has the same negative elements as the job you left. If you can pinpoint the cause of your restlessness, you may be able to solve the problem without leaving your current position. (See *Your current job: Fix it or nix it?* page 22.)

How serious are you about changing jobs?

If you're not in the job market out of necessity, are you serious about changing jobs or are you just shopping around?

YOUR CURRENT JOB: FIX IT OR NIX IT?

If you're feeling dissatisfied in your current position, think carefully before you decide to quit. Focusing on the causes of your unhappiness may help you discover possible solutions where you already work.

For instance, your discontent may stem from feeling that you're underpaid. If so, you may want to talk with your supervisor about a raise. Or you may find that you're working too many hours. Maybe you can switch to a part-time schedule. Or you may find your current position doesn't challenge you. You may want to talk with your supervisor about increasing your responsibilities or check the job listings in-house.

Keep in mind that a history of frequent job changes can harm your chances in the job market (although a job change within the same facility won't harm your chances in a future job search, as long as you weren't demoted). Potential employers want workers who show commitment. They want to hire people who have stayed at least 3 years in each position. After all, if you've left earlier jobs so readily, what will stop you from leaving the next job? A history of frequent job changes may keep you from getting to the interview stage. But if you've taken the time to think about what's making you unhappy and discover that you really can't make your current position work for you, you can proceed in your job search with confidence.

On a scale of 1 to 10, where 1 means you're not willing to change jobs and 10 means that you're very serious about accepting a new position, where would you rank yourself? Be honest. In my experience, if you rank yourself below 7, you probably won't make a change. Also, if you've been employed at the same company for more than 7 years, you probably won't leave unless you have to. If you're not serious about accepting a new position, you're wasting time and money—not only yours, but a potential employer's. And

I LIKE WHERE I AM

Susan was thrilled. She'd just received an excellent job offer, a job she really wanted a — job that meant she'd have to move. As she thought about it, reality set in. She began to feel nervous. "You know," she said to her friend, "I've had the same mailman, the same house, and the same boss for 11 years." Susan was comfortable where she was.

Change can be painful, unsettling, and downright scary. In Susan's case, she was ready to change jobs but realized she couldn't bring herself to move. And she still has that same mailman, same house, and same boss.

that's not fair to anyone. In this scenario, it took an actual job offer to make the candidate realize how much she wanted to stay put. (See *I like where I am.*)

What kind of position do you want?

Once you've determined why you're searching and that you're serious about finding a new job, you need to focus on what you want.

FIRST TIMER   If you're a student, what clinical areas might you consider? Are there specific areas you wouldn't consider? ❖

- Do you want to find a position similar to the one you currently have?
- Would you consider a different clinical specialty? For example, if you're a Critical Care Nurse but you also have a well-rounded background in medical-surgical nursing and neurology, you can readily switch to one of those areas. Or perhaps you'd be open to a Shift Supervisor position.

If you can be flexible, your opportunities will increase. However, if you're trying to break into an area where you have little or no experience, you'll have a harder time. (See chapter 1, The Preliminaries, for advice on switching clinical specialties.)

What's the most important aspect of a new job?

You've decided in general what kind of position you want. But what *specifically* do you want in a new position? To help you decide, rank the following in order of their importance to you. Feel free to add your own considerations to the list:

- salary
- location
- increased challenge and responsibility
- autonomy
- a mentor to help you transition into your new role
- the chance to work in a teaching facility
- tuition reimbursement
- supportive administration.

Ranking these factors helps you determine what a new job *must* offer and what would be "icing on the cake." For example, if you rank location first and salary third, you may accept a job that has a somewhat lower salary if it's in the right location.

What's the lowest salary you'd accept?

For the ideal job, what's the absolute lowest salary you would consider, given your current cost of living? It doesn't necessarily have to be your dream salary, but it should be a salary you could accept and be happy with. You should determine this baseline acceptable salary before you get an offer.

When could you start?

Once you have a job offer you want to accept, how much notice should you give your current employer? Most health care employers expect at least 1 month's notice, and it's never a good idea to leave without giving that much notice. First, it's not professional. Second, a potential employer may ask your references if you're eligible for rehire; if you give too little notice, you may not be. And last, but not least, giving less than a month's notice would not only leave your current employer shorthanded but would also send a message to your new employer that you might do the same thing to them.

If you must relocate, try to give yourself extra time for the move. Also, remember that you won't accrue vacation time until you've been at your new job for a while, so if you need a short break, try to build that into your time frame. Other personal considerations—such as wanting to wait for you or other family members to complete the school year—can also affect your start date. On average, you'll be expected to start around 5 to 7 weeks after receiving an offer, although you may be expected to start sooner. Few employers will want to wait more than 2 months.

Warning: Quitting your current job before you have a new position may be hazardous to your job search and career. Don't do it! (See *Don't quit now,* page 26.)

PERSONAL ASSESSMENT

If you only cared about the professional aspects of a job, you'd probably be willing to accept a position anywhere in the country—perhaps in the world—as long as that position met your professional criteria. But you can't do that. You have to think carefully about where you want to live. If you have family that would have to move with you, the task becomes even trickier.

DON'T QUIT NOW

If you're employed—even in a job you really want to leave—don't quit! You may think that quitting will give you the time you need to find a job. Or you may think it will give you that extra time to take care of family business, to relocate if you have to, or even to take a break before starting a new job. But it's harder to find a job when you're unemployed.

To potential employers, unemployment raises a red flag. Perhaps the candidate was fired, didn't get along well with coworkers, or performed poorly on the job. Potential employers are looking for "normal," and normal typically includes already having a job. As they may see it, a potential employee should want to work, not take time off; she should make good career decisions, not flighty ones like quitting a job before having a new position.

So when your résumé comes across that hiring official's desk, you don't want it to stand out because you've taken time off. Résumés that include periods of unemployment or frequent job changes tend to hit the reject pile first. A busy hiring official doesn't want to waste time on a candidate who may have potential problems. Sure, your résumé should stand out—but because it shows you're the best person for the job.

That's where the personal assessment comes in. Before you begin to search, you need to determine where you're willing to look. Can you move clear across the country? Do you want to stay near or move closer to extended family? Should you stay where you are? This section helps you and your family to think about these crucial questions. You may discover some surprising answers.

Can you relocate?

The following questions will help you decide whether you can or should relocate.

- Can you legally move out of state? Do you have to deal with a custody issue, for instance?
- Do you have college credits that won't transfer? Or is your employer paying for your education in return for a certain number of years of employment?
- Do you need to remain near aging parents?
- Will you be financially vested soon?
- Is your spouse close to retirement?
- Do you have children in their junior or senior year of high school?
- Can your spouse relocate? Is he even *willing* to relocate?
- How does the rest of your family feel about relocating?

These last two questions are among the most important. You must have the support of your family if you're all going to move. Include them in your discussions and in the decision-making process. You may need to push them hard to get to their true feelings but it's worth the effort. (See *I don't really want to go,* page 28.)

You may think of other questions to add to this list. But they should all guide you back to the most basic question: Can you relocate? If you can't, you'll have more limited options, but you'll also know where you should concentrate your efforts — close to home.

You want to relocate: What's next?

 ON THE MOVE   If you want to and can relocate, you have a new set of questions to address. First — and most important — where do you want to live? ❖

I DON'T REALLY WANT TO GO

As Director of Critical Care Nursing, Sarah made significant contributions to the hospital where she worked, and she was ready for the next step in her career. She excitedly talked with her husband, Sam, about looking for a new position, possibly one that meant moving. "If it's that important to you, I'll try to support you," he told her, a bit reluctantly. Sarah got the answer she wanted and didn't push any further.

After a few months, she received an excellent offer as Chief of Nursing at a small hospital in another state. She asked Sam what he thought about moving. "If you really want the position, I guess I'll go with you," he told her. But when push came to shove, he couldn't do it. Sarah ended up moving; Sam didn't.

Where will you move?

The list of potential questions you can ask is endless, but the following can get you started:

- What location would be your first choice?
- Where else would you consider?
- Do you have family or friends already living in a location you're considering?
- Where *won't* you go, no matter how attractive the position?
- Do you prefer urban, suburban, or rural living?
- Do you want to live in a place that has cultural activities? Proximity to golf courses or skiing? Good professional sports teams? What specific attributes are important to you?
- Do you want to be near water, mountains, or desert?
- Do you hate snow? Extreme heat?
- Do you need to live near a major airport?

- Do you care more about the location or the position it-self?

As you answer these questions and others you come up with, get yourself a map of the United States and start crossing off states that don't meet your criteria.

What problems may arise?

The possibility of relocating brings with it a slew of potential problems. The following questions can help you start planning ahead. The more planning you do, the easier relocating will be.

- Do you have school-age children? When would be the best time for them to move?
- Do you have a family member with special needs? Will the new location have the facilities necessary to meet those needs?
- Does someone in the family plan to continue his or her education? What schools, colleges, and universities does the new location have?
- Do you have pets that may make it difficult to find a place to rent?
- Do you have to sell your house? You may want to put your house on the market as soon as you decide to relocate because the chances that your house will sell and you'll accept a position at the same time are slim. If your house sells quickly, you can always store your belongings and rent while your search progresses; it's better to go through some inconvenience now than to face both mortgage and rent payments or two mortgage payments after accepting a position.
- Do you have a signed lease with your landlord? Can you shorten the lease if necessary?

- Do you need full or partial financial relocation assistance, or can you afford to move yourself?
- Will your spouse need to find a job? It's unlikely both of you will find jobs at the same time. Discuss who has the primary job and who will have the most difficulty finding a new position. Maybe the family could live on your salary while your spouse looks, or maybe your spouse could keep his job for now and follow later.

What else will affect where you might move?

Another factor in where you move is the cost of living. You should end up, not necessarily with a higher salary, but with the same or greater buying power in your new location. In some cases, you may end up with much more buying power even on a substantially lower salary.

For instance, say you live in Urbana, Illinois, and make $50,000 a year. You're considering a position in Manhattan that pays $80,000. Sounds like a good increase, doesn't it? But a comparable salary in Manhattan to the $50,000 you make in Urbana is approximately $138,000. In practical terms, you'd be taking a pay *cut*. Going the other way, if you're making $70,000 at a job in Manhattan and receive an offer of $55,000 in Urbana, you'd be looking at a pretty good increase in terms of buying power. If you don't pay attention to cost-of-living differences, you may turn down a good offer for the wrong reason. (See *Less really can be more.*)

You can obtain cost-of-living information on the Internet and from the reference section at your in public library. Because this is such an important aspect of deciding to accept a job in a new location, you might want to compare information from several sources. The following Web sites and references can lead you to the information you need. (See *Making the right move,* pages 32 and 33.)

IN REAL LIFE

LESS REALLY CAN BE MORE

Mike earned $70,000 at a hospital in the Northeast, a part of the country with a very high cost of living. The hospital was preparing to close, so Mike needed to find a new job. He interviewed for an excellent position at a hospital in the South and received an offer. But the job paid $48,000—at first glance, a big pay cut from the $70,000 Mike earned in the Northeast. Mike knew that if he took into account the difference in cost of living, the $48,000 offer would actually increase his buying power substantially. But he still had trouble taking what looked like pay cut. He told the potential employer he was making $70,000 at his current position and gave them no indication that he would accept less. He didn't hear from that employer again, even when he tried calling several times. Mike remained unemployed for more than a year.

What else do you need to do?

Breaking down the sometimes overwhelming process of relocating into specific tasks can help make it more manageable. Below you'll find some suggestions that can help you relocate.

- Contact the state board of nursing where you're planning to move for licensure information (see the appendix State Boards of Nursing) and request a licensure packet. Specific requirements depend on your area of clinical practice and your license, but you still must make sure you can practice in that state *before* you quit your current job. Find out how long it will take to receive your new license and, if necessary, get a temporary license. Some states can take as long as 3 months or more to process a license, and you'll need that license before you can practice. Some employers won't extend an offer until you have a license in

MAKING THE RIGHT MOVE

Thinking about moving? Use the following Web sites and publications to help you compare where you live now with where you're thinking of moving. Keep in mind that the cost-of-living comparisons don't take taxes into consideration. And remember to use more than one source.

Web sites

http://www.virtualrelocation.com

This site gives city-to-city comparisons of everything from average commute time to cost of living to violent crime rates. It also includes useful relocation tools that link you to information about banks, school systems, doctors, the best places to live, economic resources, available rentals, moving and storage companies, relocating with children, and much more.

http://www.homefair.com

The Salary Calculator (available in English and Spanish) at this site takes your current salary and computes how much money you'd need if you moved to any specific city. Other features include moving and mortgage-qualifying calculators, a snapshot view of different cities, and state tax tables.

http://pathfinder.com.money/bestplaces

This interesting site offers a list of the 300 best places to live in the United States, based on such data as air and water quality, crime levels, schools, and other factors. The site also helps you determine the best place for you to live by having you choose from such factors as housing, the economy, arts and culture, health, education, weather, crime, transportation, and so on. You can also use this Web page to compare the cost of living between any two U.S. cities, calculate what your mortgage would be, find an apartment, and more.

MAKING THE RIGHT MOVE *(continued)*

Publication

Each quarter, the American Chamber of Commerce Researchers Association publishes the *American Chamber of Commerce Cost of Living Index.* You can find it in your public library. The index gives the overall cost of living for a location and then breaks that down further into such categories as groceries, housing, utilities, transportation, health care, and miscellaneous goods and services. This lets you see, for example, that housing may cost 25% more in the city you're interested in, but groceries cost 15% less.

---

hand, although this is the exception, not the rule. So the earlier you start the process, the better off you'll be.

- Call the local Chamber of Commerce where you plan to move and ask for a newcomer's packet. It should contain information about housing, schools, churches, cultural activities, recreation, industry, and more. You also can find out a great deal about different communities on the Internet.

- Contact the Human Resources Department of the facility where you've applied for a position and ask if they could send you a recruitment packet. They also may be able to recommend a realtor.

- Get a copy of the local Sunday newspaper where you plan to move. It should have useful housing information and potential job opportunities for your spouse. And it can give you a good feel for the community.

YOUR BLUEPRINT

The assessment process isn't easy or quick—it's not something you can complete during lunch. It takes lots of family input, careful thought, and probably some soul-searching. But it lets you develop the blueprint you need for a successful job search. Without this blueprint, you won't know what you're really looking for and may end up with a job you hate—or with no new job at all. With this blueprint, you'll have the key to find the position you *really* want.

3

THE TOOLS

You've gone through the preliminaries and assessed what kind of position would be right for you, personally and professionally. Now you're ready to prepare the tools you need to market your background—the résumé and cover letter.

Everyone has an opinion about what to include in a résumé and cover letter. This chapter looks specifically at what works in a *nursing* résumé and cover letter and includes several examples you can use to guide you in creating your own. It also offers tips on choosing references to give to a potential employer.

THE RÉSUMÉ

A good résumé is crucial to your job search. In many cases, it's the first glimpse an employer gets of you. If it gives a bad impression, you may never be able to recover, even if you get the chance. If it gives a good impression, it can be your ticket to the interview.

What's the difference between a résumé and curriculum vitae?

A résumé and curriculum vitae (CV) serve the same purpose, but a résumé is shorter, describing a person's background in less depth than a CV. A candidate usually would need a

CV for a faculty or research position at a university. What the typical health care employer wants falls somewhere between the two. The employer wants to see all the relevant information necessary to decide if you can do the job but doesn't want everything in your background. This chapter will continue to use the word *résumé* to refer to what's really a sort of hybrid résumé-CV.

How long should a résumé be?

Common wisdom says a résumé should be no longer than two pages—but for a nursing résumé, common wisdom is wrong. A potential health care employer wants and needs to know your background in depth. What roles did you have, and what specifically did you do in those roles? Did you just do your job, or did you go beyond what was expected and really make things happen? Your résumé should have as many pages as needed to include all relevant experience.

Of course, if you're a student or have worked for only one or two employers, you may have a résumé that's only one to two pages long, and that's fine. But if you're a seasoned professional with a wealth of excellent experience that strengthens your case as the best person for the job, you'll obviously have a longer résumé. (See *Too much is a good thing.*) Nursing résumés typically range from two to five pages. But as long as you make sure that everything you've listed is relevant, the length can take care of itself.

Descriptiveness counts

When writing your résumé, describe your situation and responsibilities specifically. If you only put down your title, such as Manager of Critical Care, the potential employer won't know whether you managed a 4-bed unit open as needed with 7 employees in a 36-bed hospital or a 12-bed unit with 30 employees in a 500-bed teaching hospital. See the differ-

IN REAL LIFE

TOO MUCH IS A GOOD THING

When Michelle decided to apply for the position of Vice President of Patient Care Services at a prestigious hospital, she sent in her résumé—all 10 pages of it. A long time professional with an extensive clinical background, she needed every one of those 10 pages to present her strong clinical and progressive management experience to the potential employer, and every detail on her résumé was pertinent to the position.

Because she had not been directly involved in clinical work for some time, she also needed the longer résumé to convince the employer she would be credible to their other employees and could handle such an important position. A two-page résumé wouldn't have painted a complete picture of her but the longer résumé did, and she got the position.

ence? The hiring official may have your résumé but not the details she needs to know if you're qualified. And she won't go to the trouble to find out—she doesn't have the time! You may be the most qualified candidate for the position, but if that doesn't come through in every line of your résumé, you may not even get an interview.

It's up to you to paint a clear and complete picture of your background, one that will catch a hiring official's eye and keep her from weeding out your résumé. Show her who you are professionally, where you've been, and what you've done. Emphasize those aspects of your background that make you the best candidate. Take the time to create a great first impression.

FIRST TIMER   Students, you'll need to mention every bit of pertinent experience from your background, including clinical rotations, to show a potential employer why you deserve another look. Specifics will increase your chances of being hired. ❖

General guidelines

The following tips can help you create the best résumé:

- Use only quality, 24-lb, white or cream-colored paper. The employer will probably make copies of your résumé for everyone on the interview schedule, and white or cream-colored paper copies best. Shaded or dark paper is a copying nightmare, and any border or patterned paper you choose won't suit everyone. You want the employer to judge you on your qualifications, not on your taste in stationery.

- Prepare your résumé on a computer, not a typewriter. A résumé prepared on a typewriter can give the employer the impression that you're not flexible and can't keep pace with changes in technology. You can choose from many popular word-processing programs, including Microsoft Word or WordPerfect, or you can use a software program specifically designed for résumé preparation. Print your résumé on a laser printer for crisp, clear copies.

- Use a 10- to 12-point font size; smaller fonts are difficult to read, especially when copied.

- If you opt for a résumé preparation service, tell them explicitly what you want. Such services typically prepare business résumés, not nursing résumés.

- List your positions, education, and so forth in reverse chronological order, beginning with the most recent.

- Don't include personal information on your résumé, such as age, marital status, religion, race, color, national origin, health status, children, or disabilities. Don't include names of organizations or scholarships, such as Minority Health Profession, that would reveal any of this information. And don't enclose a photo.

- Don't mention your current, most recent, or required salary on your résumé.

- Don't list continuing education units.

- Just as you would in a patient assessment, keep the information you supply objective. For example, don't write that you work in "a busy emergency department"; what you consider busy may differ drastically from what the employer considers busy. Instead, write that you work in "an emergency department that sees 50,000 patients a year."
- Make sure your résumé has absolutely, positively no typographic or spelling errors. A hiring official faced with a stack of résumés may reason that someone who overlooks such an error wouldn't make a conscientious employee, and she'll use that typo to weed out your résumé. So triple-check your résumé; then have at least one other person read through it again.
- Never, ever lie on your résumé. Remember, exaggerating is lying. Honesty is the best policy—in fact, it's the only policy. Lying on a résumé or application is grounds for dismissal.
- Maintain a 1" margin at the top, bottom, and sides of your résumé. Cramming too much on a page makes it difficult to read. Instead, use as many pages as you need to make your résumé legible and easy to read. Use a triple space between sections, a double space after headings, and a single space between paragraphs.
- Don't use hyphens at the end of a line when a word is too long. Go to the next line to begin the word instead.
- Put your name on every page of your résumé. An employer may receive many résumés, and a page can easily be misplaced.
- Number the pages of your résumé, starting with page two.
- Don't staple your résumé; it makes it harder to copy.
- Don't write on your résumé for any reason.
- If you have to fax your résumé to a potential employer, mail out a hard copy the same day.

- Don't fold your cover letter and résumé when you mail them. Instead, use a page-size envelope.
- Make sure you use enough postage; the larger envelopes usually take extra postage. An employer won't look kindly on having to pay to pick up your résumé at the post office!
- Keep an accurate record of every résumé you mail, including the date you sent it, the name of the person and company you sent it to, any response you received, and when and what you did to follow up.

Creating your résumé — step-by-step

A résumé has several standard sections, including heading, objective (this section is optional but recommended), education, professional experience, certification and licensures, professional affiliations, honors and awards, presentations, and research and publications. If you wish, you can finish with a line about available references.

Heading

Your résumé begins with the heading. The first line should include your name; the next, your street address; and the third, your city, state, and zip code.

The fourth line should list your home phone number, including area code. As soon as you've put your home phone number on your résumé, make sure that the message on your answering machine or voice mail sounds professional. Don't use a "cute" message, and avoid background music. You also can include your work number but only if you don't mind a potential employer calling you at work. You may not want to include it if anyone else might answer your phone or if your voice mail isn't confidential.

A final line can include your E-mail address. Don't list it if confidentiality is a problem or if the address sounds unprofessional — hotlips@mail.net, for example.

Objective

A good objective should be brief, just one or two sentences to state your position goal. Although it's optional, a well-worded objective can really help. Without it, a hiring official must read through your entire résumé to determine what you're qualified for. With it, she can quickly determine that you may be just what they're looking for and shoot your résumé over to the "must contact" pile.

If you're flexible about the position you want, you can write a general objective, such as "To obtain a challenging management or supervisory position." Or you can tailor the objective on each résumé to a specific position you know to be available, such as "To obtain a Nurse-Manager position on a telemetry unit" or "To obtain a Nurse-Manager position on a medical-surgical unit."

Education

You can include education here or after professional experience, depending on your situation. You should include your education here if you:

 FIRST TIMER   are a new RN graduate ❖

- have a strong educational background for the position you seek
- have at least a master's degree
- want a staff position and have little or no experience
- want a position other than staff, such as Nurse-Manager, Case Manager, or Staff Educator, and have a bachelor's degree or higher.

Include your education *after* your professional experience if you:

- have the experience the employer wants but don't have the preferred or required education; this builds on your strengths by making sure the potential employer sees your experience before getting to your education

- want a position such as Director of Nursing, Chief Nursing Officer, or Vice President of Nursing or Patient Care Services and have a diploma, associate's degree, or bachelor's degree
- want a position other than staff, such as Nurse-Manager, Case Manager, or Staff Educator, and have a diploma or associate's degree.

Wherever you place your education, the first line should include the university you attended, including city and state. The next line should list the degree and focus of the program and the year you received or expect to receive your degree. Don't include your high-school education.

Professional experience

Your professional experience should begin with the month (or quarter if you're a student) and year you worked at a facility, followed by the name of the facility, including city and state. Next should come your title and your responsibilities and accomplishments.

 FIRST TIMER   If you're a new graduate and have worked in nursing while in school, include part-time or full-time work here and describe your responsibilities and accomplishments. ❖

When recording responsibilities, be specific and descriptive, and use action verbs. (See *Action verbs.*) Avoid starting sentences with the word "I." Identify your specific responsibilities, such as direct patient care, budgeting, hiring, firing, staffing, and 24-hour accountability. Specify the type and number of units or areas of the facility where you worked, the number of employees you managed, and any research or staff, patient, or family education you performed. Include working as a student preceptor, performing evaluations, acting as charge nurse, working in inpatient or outpatient areas, performing quality assurance, preparing critical pathways,

ACTION VERBS

Using action verbs can really make your responsibilities and accomplishments stand out. Choose from the following verbs when writing your résumé and cover letter.

Accomplished	Compiled	Diagnosed
Achieved	Completed	Diagrammed
Acted	Composed	Directed
Administered	Computed	Discovered
Advanced	Conceived	Dispensed
Advised	Concentrated	Displayed
Analyzed	Conceptualized	Distributed
Anticipated	Condensed	Diverted
Applied	Conducted	Doubled
Appointed	Conserved	Downsized
Approved	Consolidated	Drafted
Arbitrated	Constructed	Earned
Arranged	Contacted	Edited
Assembled	Controlled	Eliminated
Assessed	Converted	Employed
Assisted	Coordinated	Enforced
Assumed	Corrected	Ensured
Attained	Corresponded	Established
Audited	Counseled	Estimated
Authored	Cowrote	Evaluated
Broadened	Created	Examined
Budgeted	Cut	Executed
Built	Decentralized	Exhibited
Calculated	Decreased	Expanded
Centralized	Defined	Expedited
Certified	Delegated	Explained
Chaired	Delivered	Explored
Coached	Demonstrated	Facilitated
Coauthored	Designed	Filed
Cochaired	Detailed	Focused
Collaborated	Determined	Formed
Collected	Developed	Formulated
Combined	Devised	Founded
Communicated	Devoted	

(continued)

ACTION VERBS *(continued)*

Gathered	Mediated	Raised
Generated	Merged	Read
Guaranteed	Met	Realized
Guided	Minimized	Received
Handled	Modified	Recommended
Headed	Monitored	Recorded
Helped	Motivated	Recruited
Hired	Negotiated	Redesigned
Identified	Observed	Reduced
Illustrated	Obtained	Referred
Implemented	Offered	Regulated
Improved	Operated	Rehabilitated
Increased	Ordered	Reinforced
Influenced	Organized	Related
Informed	Originated	Renegotiated
Initiated	Overhauled	Reorganized
Innovated	Participated	Reported
Inspected	Passed	Repositioned
Installed	Performed	Represented
Instituted	Persuaded	Reproduced
Instructed	Planned	Researched
Integrated	Practiced	Reshaped
Interpreted	Predicted	Resolved
Interviewed	Prepared	Responded
Introduced	Prescribed	Restored
Invented	Presented	Restructured
Investigated	Prevented	Retrieved
Justified	Printed	Revamped
Launched	Processed	Reversed
Lectured	Programmed	Reviewed
Led	Projected	Revised
Located	Promoted	Revitalized
Lowered	Proposed	Saved
Maintained	Protected	Scheduled
Managed	Proved	Screened
Marketed	Provided	Selected
Maximized	Publicized	Served
Measured	Published	Set

ACTION VERBS *(continued)*

Showed	Succeeded	Treated
Simplified	Summarized	Tripled
Solved	Superseded	Uncovered
Sought	Supervised	Undertook
Spearheaded	Supplied	Unified
Specified	Supported	United
Spoke	Sustained	Updated
Staffed	Taught	Used
Standardized	Terminated	Utilized
Started	Tracked	Validated
Streamlined	Trained	Verified
Strengthened	Transferred	Won
Stressed	Transformed	Worked
Structured	Translated	Wrote
Studied	Traveled	

working in case management, or anything else that might be relevant. Don't copy information from your job description.

When listing accomplishments, again, be specific and descriptive and use action verbs. Whenever you can, include objective observations and numbers. Did you save the organization money? How much? Did you help it make money? How much? Were you involved in starting up a unit? In downsizing or moving to a new facility? Do you have experience in program development or have you handled any special projects? Did you help develop policies and procedures, a continuous quality improvement program, critical pathways, or outreach programs? Have you taken part in team building?

All these accomplishments add to your résumé, so take the time you need to compile this information, and be thorough. You'll use this information again in your cover letter and during your interview.

Other information you may want to list under professional experience include:

- any special knowledge or skills you have, such as computer skills
- the title — but not the name — of the person to whom you reported in each position
- the number of beds in the facility where you worked
- the type of facility, such as teaching, pediatric, oncology, surgery center, hospice, health maintenance organization, family practice clinic, level I trauma center, urgent care center, or dialysis center; mention if the facility is union or nonunion and for-profit or nonprofit.

Some final tips: Don't mention non-nursing experience on your résumé. Also, if you worked at the same facility more than once, list both times together so the employer — who may only have time to glance at your résumé — doesn't get the impression you're a job hopper. Make it easy for the employer. And don't forget: If it isn't on your résumé, you haven't done it.

Certifications and licensures

Include only nursing certifications and licensures, and list only valid certifications (the expiration date is optional); employers aren't interested in certifications that are no longer current. However, you should list all licensures, active or inactive. Note the type of license, number, state, and expiration date. Include any examinations you're scheduled to take, including the type of examination and date.

Professional affiliations

Like certifications and licensures, professional affiliations must be related to nursing. Examples you should list include the National Student Nurses Association; the Oncology Nursing Society; and the Wound, Ostomy, and Continence Nurses Society.

Honors and awards

List any special awards or honors that you've received. Such honors tell a potential employer that you've been recognized for working hard and performing well—in fact, for doing more than expected. That's the kind of employee they want working for them. Such honors may include Dean's List or Employee of the Year.

Presentations

List only pertinent nursing-related presentations, and include the title, audience, and date. These presentations should show the employer that you've gone beyond the call of duty, have done more than the average person on the job, and have a sense of commitment.

 FIRST TIMER   Students, if you've given a nursing-related presentation during a clinical rotation to your nursing class, or to any other organization, include those here. ❖

Research and publications

List only pertinent nursing-related research. Include all researchers' names, the title of the project, and the date. Also, list only pertinent nursing-related publications; include the title, publication, and date.

References on request

It's up to you whether or not you want to end your résumé with a line about references being available on request. Of course, you'll provide references, but you shouldn't list the actual references on your résumé. Doing so may make potential employers feel obliged to call your references, and you don't want your references inconvenienced by every person who receives your résumé.

Sample résumés

The following sections examine sample résumés from a Student Nurse, Staff Nurse, Clinical Nurse Specialist, Nurse Practitioner, Director of Nursing, and Vice President of Nursing. (See *Sample résumés,* pages 49 to 53, 55 to 61, and 63 to 69.) They can serve as guidelines for putting together your résumé.

Student Nurse résumé

FIRST TIMER   This résumé from a student includes a general objective that applies to positions in any clinical area. With no real work experience as an RN, the author lists her education first. She records her clinical rotations next, followed by her current job as a Nursing Assistant. This lets the employer see her first as an RN but also shows that she has additional patient care experience. She uses quarter/year for dates, switching to month/year for her current position. Under certification, she notes when she's scheduled to take the NCLEX examination. ❖

From this résumé, a prospective employer might conclude that Jane:
- values quality patient care, as stated in the objective
- would make a committed, responsible employee, as evidenced by her Dean's List standing and nursing scholarship
- has a good idea of what she's getting into because she has worked as a Nursing Assistant.

Staff Nurse résumé

The clear objective in this Staff Nurse's résumé lets the employer know up front that the author seeks a position in rehabilitation. Bren's strong rehabilitation clinical experience outweighs his educational background, so he lists his professional experience first. Notice how he gives the most detail about his rehabilitation position. The employer can also see that Bren is pursuing a bachelor's degree while working,

(Text continues on page 54.)

STUDENT NURSE RÉSUMÉ

Jane Zanski
4848 West Apprentice Way
Owensboro, Kentucky 42301
(502) 364-5555

OBJECTIVE

To obtain a challenging RN position where I can use and enhance my knowledge and skills to provide quality patient care.

EDUCATION

Waldon University, Paducah, Kentucky
Bachelor of Science in Nursing, expected 5/99

STUDENT CLINICAL EXPERIENCE

Spring/99
Acute Care Rotation
Foust Medical Center, Paducah, Kentucky
250-bed acute care facility. Clinical rotations on medical/surgical unit, OR, medical/surgical ICU, ED, and orthopedic units.

Psychiatric Rotation
Veterans Administration Hospital, Owensboro, Kentucky
400-bed acute care facility. Clinical rotation involving patients in geropsych and a locked adult psychiatric ward.

Fall/98
Obstetric and Pediatric Rotation
Christian Hospital for Women and Children, Bowling Green, Kentucky
150-bed facility. Clinical rotations on antepartum, labor and delivery, postpartum, newborn nursery, and pediatric units.

Spring/98
Chronic Care Rotation
Hopewell Manor, Whitesville, Kentucky
100-bed long-term care facility. Clinical rotations in long-term care, rehabilitation, and hospice. Volunteered to assist with home health patients.

(continued)

STUDENT NURSE RÉSUMÉ *(continued)*

Jane Zanski
page 2

WORK EXPERIENCE

1/96-Present
Nursing Assistant, Medical/Surgical Unit
Blue Ridge Hospital, Owensboro, Kentucky
120-bed community hospital. Perform direct patient care on a 32-bed
medical/surgical unit. Responsibilities include obtaining patient assessments,
assisting with activities of daily living, and maintaining patients' safety.
Report to Charge Nurse.

CERTIFICATIONS/LICENSURES

*   Basic Cardiac Life Support
*   NCLEX examination scheduled, 6/99

HONORS/AWARDS

*   Dean's List, Waldon University, 12/98
*   Blue Ridge Hospital Nursing Scholarship, 6/96

REFERENCES

Available upon request

STAFF NURSE RÉSUMÉ

BREN JORDAN
444 South Vine, #3B
Owensboro, Kentucky 42301
(502) 685-1783

OBJECTIVE

To obtain a challenging position in rehabilitation nursing where I can use my clinical knowledge and experience.

PROFESSIONAL EXPERIENCE

5/95-present **United Hospital,** Owensboro, Kentucky
300-bed teaching facility

Staff RN, Rehabilitation Unit
Responsibilities on a 30-bed inpatient rehabilitation unit include performing direct patient care, conducting assessments, organizing floor in-service workshops, and facilitating patient and family education. Serve as skin care advisor in prevention and treatment of decubiti. Cases include cerebrovascular accident, head and spinal cord injury, hip/knee replacement, amputee, multiple trauma, and general debility patients. Report to Program Director.

2/92-3/95 **Memorial Hospital,** Ottumwa, Iowa
250-bed community hospital

Staff RN, Telemetry Unit
Provided primary nursing care to medical and surgical patients requiring telemetry monitoring on a 16-bed unit. Primarily consisted of cardiac and postsurgical patients. Reported to Nurse Manager.

6/86-12/91 **Community Hospital,** Salida, Colorado
80-bed community hospital

Staff RN, Medical/Surgical Unit
Performed nursing care for a variety of medical/surgical patients, including COPD, oncology, HIV, hospice, and CVA patients. Reported to Head Nurse.

(continued)

BREN JORDAN
Page 2

6/84-5/86   **Office of Edmond Hughes, M.D.,** Ottumwa, Iowa
Family practice clinic

Office Nurse
Prepared patients for examination, completed assessments,
obtained histories, monitored patient medications, ordered
supplies, and sterilized instruments. Created patient and
family education program. Reported to physician.

9/81-5/84   **Doctors Hospital,** Oak Ridge, Tennessee
150-bed community hospital

Nursing Assistant, Medical/Surgical Unit
Performed direct patient care on a 32-bed medical/surgical
unit.

EDUCATION

University College, Owensboro, Kentucky
Bachelor of Business degree, expected 6/99

Indian Hills Community College, Ottumwa, Iowa
Associate of Science in Nursing, 5/86

Indian Hills Community College, Centerville, Iowa
Licensed Practical Nurse Program, 6/84

CERTIFICATIONS

- Certified Rehabilitation RN
- Basic Cardiac Life Support
- Advanced Cardiac Life Support

LICENSURES

- LPN #33-3333B, Iowa, inactive
- RN #555-555555A, Iowa, inactive
- RN #333-333333A, Colorado, expires 5/00
- RN #222-222222A, Kentucky, expires 9/99

BREN JORDAN
Page 3

PROFESSIONAL AFFILIATIONS

- Association of Rehabilitation Nurses
- American Nurses Association
- Student Nurses Association
- Kentucky Nurses Association

HONORS/AWARDS

- Memorial Hospital Employee of the Month, 7/94
- President of RN Nursing Class, Indian Hills Community College, 1986
- Graduated with honors, 4.0 GPA, 5/86
- E.E. Martin Memorial Nursing Scholarship, 5/85
- Doctors Hospital Nursing Scholarship, 6/83

PRESENTATIONS

- "CRRN: The Benefits," Kentucky Rehabilitation Conference, 9/98
- "Preparation for JCAHO and CARF Accreditations," Indiana Rehabilitation Conference, 5/97
- "Rehabilitation: The Long Road Home," Students Against Drunk Driving, Owensboro High School, 4/97
- "Spinal Cord Injury," University College Department of Nursing, 10/96
- "Care of the Brain Injured Patient," United Hospital Inservice, 6/96

REFERENCES

Available upon request

showing that he still wants to grow professionally. Bren next includes certifications and licensures, and then professional affiliations, honors, and presentations that relate to rehabilitation. What doesn't—and shouldn't—appear on this résumé is Bren's nonnursing part-time job at a restaurant.

Clinical Nurse Specialist résumé

The very specific objective in this résumé, narrowed not only to oncology but to Clinical Nurse Specialist in pediatric oncology, lets the employer know exactly what Patricia wants in a position. The author lists her strong educational background first and then highlights her pediatric, oncology, and Clinical Nurse Specialist responsibilities in the section on experience. She next includes appropriate certifications and affiliations, honors and awards, and presentations and research, giving further proof that she can do the job.

An employer looking for a Clinical Nurse Specialist needs a good resource person for the specific specialty, someone who can be the authority in that clinical area and handle the research that is part of the job. Patricia's in-depth résumé shows that she's well qualified in all these areas and can readily fill the position.

Nurse Practitioner résumé

Like the Clinical Nurse Specialist résumé, this résumé includes a very specific objective. The strong education is listed first, especially because Shirley hasn't actually worked as a Nurse Practitioner and her clinical rotations weren't related to oncology. Notice how she groups her clinical duties as a Student Nurse Practitioner together and then goes into detail describing her strong oncology background. She then includes her licensure and scheduled certification examination as well as other pertinent certifications, affiliations, awards, presen-

(Text continues on page 62.)

CLINICAL NURSE SPECIALIST RÉSUMÉ

Patricia Herrera
8080 North Parkway South, #434
Alamosa, Colorado 81101
(719) 589-5555
email: pherrera@talk.net

OBJECTIVE

To practice as an Oncology Clinical Nurse Specialist in a pediatric setting.

EDUCATION

University of Salida, Salida, Colorado
Doctorate of Science in Nursing, Nursing/Research, Pediatric Oncology, 5/98

Alamosa College, Alamosa, Colorado
Master of Science in Nursing, Clinical Nurse Specialist, Oncology focus, 12/93

University of Leadville, Leadville, Colorado
Bachelor of Science in Nursing, 5/89
GPA 4.0

Major Hospital School of Nursing, Alamosa, Colorado
Nursing diploma, 5/81

**PROFESSIONAL
EXPERIENCE
6/94-Present**

Major Hospital, Alamosa, Colorado
300-bed regional referral center

Clinical Nurse Specialist, Oncology
Serve as resource person for both an18-bed oncology unit and outpatient areas. Collaborate with management, physicians, hospital administration, nursing managers, and ancillary units. Responsibilities include staff, patient, and family education; program development; coordination of preceptor and orientation experiences; research; case management; and quality assurance. Patients include children and adults. Report to Director of Nursing.

(continued)

CLINICAL NURSE SPECIALIST RÉSUMÉ *(continued)*

Herrera, Patricia
page 2

6/90-5/94
Blessing Medical Center, Alamosa, Colorado
200-bed acute care facility

Nurse Manager, Oncology Unit
Maintained 24-hour accountability for a 12-bed oncology
unit, including 20 full-time employees. Hired and fired staff;
developed and administered budget; counseled, disciplined, and
evaluated employees; and conducted staff education. Reported to
Director of Medical/Surgical Nursing. (11/91-5/94)

Staff Nurse, Oncology Unit
Provided primary nursing care for adult and pediatric oncology
patients on 12-bed unit. Reported to Nurse Manager.
(6/90-11/91)

6/86-5/90
Hospital of Medicine, Leadville, Colorado
230-bed acute care facility

Staff Nurse, Medical/Surgical Unit
Staff Nurse, General Pediatric Unit, P.R.N.
Responsible for direct patient care on 36-bed medical/surgical
unit. Floated to 10-bed pediatric unit when necessary. Reported
to Charge Nurse.

3/84-5/86
Hope Hospital, Hope City, Tennessee
60-bed community hospital

Staff Nurse, Medical/Surgical Unit
Performed direct patient care on 36-bed medical/surgical unit.
Reported to Charge Nurse.

5/81-2/84
Crawfordsville Medical Center, Crawfordsville, Indiana
200-bed community hospital

**Staff Nurse, General Pediatric and Pediatric
Intensive Care Units**
Performed direct patient care for pediatric patients on 8-bed
general pediatric and 4-bed pediatric intensive care units.
Reported to Nurse Manager.

CLINICAL NURSE SPECIALIST RÉSUMÉ *(continued)*

Herrera, Patricia
page 3

LICENSURE

- RN license #33-55555A, Colorado, expires 10/99
- RN license #1952-25A, Tennessee, expires 6/00
- RN license #31757B, Indiana, expires 12/99

CERTIFICATIONS

- Oncology Certified Nurse
- Chemotherapy Certified
- Clinical Nurse Specialist — Oncology
- Pediatric Oncology Certification
- Basic Cardiac Life Support
- Pediatric Advanced Life Support

PROFESSIONAL
AFFILIATIONS

- Oncology Nursing Society
- American Nurses Association
- Colorado Nurses Association
- American Cancer Society
- Sigma Theta Tau National Honor Society

HONORS/AWARDS

- American Cancer Society Excellence in Cancer Award, 8/97
- National Institutes of Health, National Center for Nursing Research, Director's Award, 6/97
- Fellow of the American Academy of Nursing, 6/96
- President, Nursing Class, Alamosa College, 92-93
- Employee of the Year, Blessing Medical Center, 12/92
- Oncology Foundation Scholarship, 6/91
- Sigma Theta Tau, 5/89
- National Endowment for the Humanities Summer Fellowship, University of Leadville, 6/88
- Major Hospital School of Nursing, Mary J. Knapp Scholastic Award for Outstanding Achievement, 5/81

(continued)

CLINICAL NURSE SPECIALIST RÉSUMÉ *(continued)*

Herrera, Patricia
page 4

PRESENTATIONS

- "Pain Management," Denver Nursing Conference, 8/98
- "Coping With Cancer," Colorado Jaycees, 11/97
- "Care of the Radiation Therapy Patient," Major Hospital, 3/96
- "Prostate Cancer," Blessing Medical Center, 4/94
- "Cancer: Knowledge and Attitudes," Southcentral Colorado Chapter, Oncology Nursing Society, 6/93
- "Oncology Nursing," Alamosa College of Nursing, 10/89
- "Multiple Myeloma," Leadville College of Nursing, 4/89
- "Pancreatic Cancer," Leadville Nurses' Annual Conference, 2/88

RESEARCH

- Herrera, P.A., "Patient-focused satisfaction: A comparison of general oncologic and hospice care settings," 6/97
- Herrera, P.A., "The spouse: Study of the home caregiver," 10/95

PUBLICATIONS

- "Oncology News," *Alamosa Journal-Review,* 4/98
- "Death and Dying," *Nurse Network,* 1/98
- "Preventing Colon Cancer," *The Diet Monitor,* 1/97
- "Coping with Cancer," *RN Today,* 4/96
- "Patience with Patients," *RN Today,* 11/95
- "Cancer Through the Eyes of a Child," *The Pediatric Review,* 6/95

REFERENCES

Provided upon request

Nurse Practitioner Résumé

SHIRLEY ROYBAL
4741 Rocky Knob Lane
Oak Ridge, Tennessee 37830
(423) 483-5555

OBJECTIVE
To obtain a challenging position as an Adult Nurse Practitioner in a dynamic oncology and hematology environment.

EDUCATION
Oak Ridge College, Oak Ridge, Tennessee
Master of Science in Nursing
Adult Nurse Practitioner Program, expected *6/99*

Clinton University, Clinton, Tennessee
Bachelor of Science in Nursing, *5/83*

PROFESSIONAL EXPERIENCE
8/97-Present
East Tennessee Area Hospital and Clinics, Oak Ridge, Tennessee
Adult Nurse Practitioner Student
Perform histories and physicals, provide primary care nursing, write medical orders, and interpret diagnostic tests. Authored patient education pamphlets with emphasis on health promotion and disease prevention.

5/95-Present
Compton Medical Center, Hematology/Oncology Group,
Compton Cancer Center, Oak Ridge, Tennessee
400-bed regional referral center
Staff Nurse, Hematology/Oncology
Responsible for direct patient care on 20-bed hematology/oncology medical inpatient unit and outpatient clinic. Administer chemotherapy, perform assessments, monitor adverse events, and provide pain management and family and patient education. Act as student preceptor. Report to Nurse Manager.

(continued)

SHIRLEY ROYBAL
page 2

1/91-4/95
Miracle Hospital, Clinton, Tennessee
150-bed community hospital
Staff Nurse, Oncology
Provided nursing care for oncology patients on 14-bed unit. Performed staff education and acted as Charge Nurse when necessary. Reported to Unit Supervisor.

11/86-12/90
Christian Hospital, Clinton, Tennessee
200-bed acute care facility
Staff Nurse, Telemetry
Provided primary nursing care for medical/surgical patients on 20-bed unit requiring telemetry monitoring. Conducted in-service workshops for staff nurses. Served as quality assurance committee member from unit. Assumed charge nurse duties when necessary. Reported to Head Nurse.

8/83-11/86
Hope Hospital, Hope City, Tennessee
60-bed community hospital
Staff Nurse, Medical/Surgical
Provided direct patient care on 36-bed medical/surgical unit. Rotated to intensive care and pediatric units on weekends. Assumed Charge Nurse duties when necessary. Reported to Head Nurse.

LICENSURE
• RN license #5550-20202, Tennessee, expires *10/99*

CERTIFICATIONS
• Adult Nurse Practitioner examination, scheduled *10/99*
• Oncology Certified Nurse
• Chemotherapy Certified

SHIRLEY ROYBAL
page 3

PROFESSIONAL AFFILIATIONS
- Oncology Nursing Society
- American Nurses Association
- Tennessee Nurses Association
- American Cancer Society

HONORS/AWARDS
- Oak Ridge College, Sigma Theta Tau, *12/98*
- Dean's List with distinction, *5/98*
- Dean's List, *5/97*
- American Cancer Society Graduate Scholarship in Nursing, *6/96*

PRESENTATIONS
- "Pain Management," Nashville Nursing Conference, *7/98*
- "Pain Guidelines," Compton Medical Center, *3/98*
- "Cancer: Knowledge and Attitudes," Eastern Tennessee Chapter, Oncology Nursing Society, *5/97*
- "Morphine Myths," Oak Ridge College of Nursing, *5/96*
- "Skin Cancer: An Ounce of Prevention," Oak Ridge Nurses' Annual Conference, *3/96*
- "Oncology Nursing," Oak Ridge College, *11/95*
- "Smoking: Where There's Smoke, There's Fire," Oak Ridge High School, *10/95*

PUBLICATIONS
- "Oncology Care in the Community," *Oak Ridge Register, 11/98*
- "Assessing Cancer Pain," *Today's Nurse, 4/98*
- "Cancer Prevention," *Lady's Home Journal, 3/97*
- "Breast Cancer Prevention and Treatment," *Today's Woman, 7/95*

tations, and publications, all building a strong case for Shirley to the employer. Can she do the job? Her résumé says yes.

Director of Nursing résumé

Many candidates for Director of Nursing positions have master's degrees; Vanessa doesn't. But she does have strong experience, so she has listed her professional experience before her education. Putting her impressive work history first should keep the employer from passing over her résumé based on her lack of advanced education. Vanessa brings to the forefront both the clinical expertise and managerial background employers look for in a Director of Nursing candidate.

Note that Vanessa worked at Wellness Hospital two separate times but listed them together under the hospital's name. This prevents the employer from, at first glance, thinking Vanessa worked for two different employers. It also shows that Vanessa was a good enough employee for the same hospital to hire twice — a plus for the candidate.

The bullets make this résumé easy to read, saving the employer time. Vanessa also describes her accomplishments concretely; she increased revenues by $250,000 and decreased registry use by 90%. Explaining that Cape Health Medical Center and Wellness Hospital merged lets a potential employer know why the author took a position with less responsibility and why she's looking for increased responsibility. She also groups together staff nursing positions from years ago; they won't help much in her current search, and mentioning them only briefly saves the employer unnecessary reading.

Vice President résumé

This résumé shows the author's progression from staff nurse through the levels of management to Vice President, with an increase in responsibility at each step. She discusses her Staff Nurse and Manager positions but goes into much greater

(Text continues on page 70.)

DIRECTOR OF NURSING RÉSUMÉ

VANESSA CHU
708 Old Stone Road, #1-B
Centerville, Tennessee 37033
(931) 729-5555
E-mail: vchu45@iquest.com

OBJECTIVE
To obtain a position as Director of Emergency Services with increased
challenge and responsibility.

PROFESSIONAL EXPERIENCE
8/88-Present
Wellness Hospital, Centerville, Tennessee
200-bed acute care facility

Nurse Manager, Emergency Department *(4/93-Present)*
Staff Nurse, Emergency Department *(8/88-4/93)*
Maintain 24-hour accountability for ED receiving 20,000 patients/year.
Responsibilities include budgeting, hiring, firing, staffing, evaluations, staff
education, and management of 20 full-time employees. Report to Director of
Nursing.
- Planned and supervised renovation of emergency department and addition of
  5 rooms.
- Increased customer satisfaction survey numbers by 52%.
- Created initial Continuous Quality Improvement program.
- Developed triage system.
- Revised patient flow through ED, decreasing patient wait time.
- Coordinated physician quality assurance program.
- Launched development of trauma program.
- Organized fast-track clinic through University of Centerville.
- Negotiated contract with emergency medical services in city of Centerville,
  increasing ED revenue by $250,000.
- Served as active member of Continuous Quality Improvement, utilization
  review, and product line committees.
- Organized development of citywide disaster plan.
- Spearheaded clinical career ladder for nursing department.
- Decreased registry use by 90%.
- Functioned as mentor for new managers.
- Assisted in planning and implementing housewide computerized inpatient
  documentation system.

(continued)

VANESSA CHU
Page 2

12/84-7/88
Cape Health Medical Center, Centerville, Tennessee
(Merged with Wellness Hospital *8/88*)
275-bed acute care facility

Director of Emergency Services
Maintained 24-hour accountability for ED in 275-bed acute care facility
receiving 24,000 patients/year. Responsibilities included budgeting, hiring,
firing, staffing, and evaluations for 35 full-time employees. Reported to Vice
President of Patient Services.
• Conducted in-service education.
• Directed merger of two EDs.
• Created and instituted comprehensive triage program.
• Developed and revised policies and procedures and standards of care.
• Devised comprehensive Continuous Quality Improvement plan.
• Increased number of staff certified in emergency nursing to100%.
• Assisted in redesigning and planning new ED and outpatient areas.
• Devised and implemented ED patient satisfaction survey.
• Served on JCAHO preparation task force and trauma services and
  community health services committees.

9/81-11/84
Harmless Medical Center, Centerville, Tennessee
70-bed community hospital

Staff Nurse, Emergency Department
• Performed direct patient care in ED receiving 10,000 patients/year.
• Functioned as preceptor for student nurses and new employee orientation.
• Acted as Charge Nurse on 3 to 11 shift.

5/76-7/81
Various Staff Nurse Positions
Medical/surgical units and emergency departments

EDUCATION
University of Centerville, Centerville, Tennessee
Bachelor of Science in Nursing, *12/84*

Hills Community College, Albia, Tennessee
Associate of Science in Nursing, *5/80*

VANESSA CHU
Page 3

St. Joseph Hospital School of Nursing, Centerville, Tennessee
Diploma, *5/76*

CERTIFICATIONS/LICENSURES
- RN license #000-000-000, Tennessee, expires *10/99*
- Certified Emergency Nurse, expires *3/00*
- Trauma Nurse Core Curriculum, expires *9/99*
- Advanced Cardiac Life Support Provider, expires *4/00*
- Pediatric Advanced Life Support Instructor, expires *12/99*
- Certified Flight Registered Nurse, expires *10/00*
- Pediatric Emergency Care Course Provider, expires *5/99*

PROFESSIONAL AFFILIATIONS
- Tennessee Emergency Medical Services Association
- Tennessee Trauma Society
- President, Emergency Nurses Association, 1996
- Tennessee Organization of Nurse Executives
- American Trauma Society

HONORS/AWARDS
- Chosen Nurse of the Year, Cape Health Medical Center, 12/87
- Community Volunteer of the Year, Albia Chamber of Commerce, 7/79

PRESENTATIONS
- "Emergency Room: Feast or Famine," National Emergency Nurses' General Assembly, 10/98
- "Emergency Nurses Traumatized," Emergency Nurses Association, 10/97
- "The ER: How Safe Is It?" Emergency Medicine Conference, 4/96

PUBLICATIONS
- "Emergency Nurses Traumatized," *Journal of ER,* 6/98
- "Assault in the ER," *Nursing Today,* 10/95
- "Are You Safe in the ER?," *ER Medicine,* 4/93
- "Violence in the ER," *Nursing Today,* 7/87
- "Patient Satisfaction: Are You Doing Your Part?" *Nursing Management,* 6/85

VICE PRESIDENT RÉSUMÉ

CORBIN JENKINS

2204 Sandollar Boulevard
Navarre, Florida 32566
(850) 939-5555

OBJECTIVE

To obtain a Vice President–level position in a large teaching facility.

EDUCATION

University of Florida, Navarre, Florida
Master of Business Administration, 5/87
Master of Science in Nursing, 12/84

Florida College, Navarre, Florida
Bachelor of Science in Nursing, 6/77

Saint Elizabeth Hospital School of Nursing, Andrew, Florida
Diploma in Nursing, 5/70

PROFESSIONAL EXPERIENCE

2/94-Present

Central Hospital, Navarre, Florida
Vice President of Patient Care Services
Responsible for nursing department, emergency services,
ambulatory care, surgical services (8 suites), rehabilitation,
pharmacy, and pain management in 300-bed facility with a total
of 480 full-time employees. Report to Hospital Administrator.
* Established Center for Nursing Excellence.
* Spearheaded outpatient oncology program.
* Designed and implemented the total quality management
  program.
* Transformed pharmacy department cost-reduction plan and
  enhanced productivity.
* Developed product line for cardiology.
* Reorganized nursing department, eliminating 30 full-time
  employees and saving $500,000.
* Provided plan and leadership for restructuring facility into
  patient-focused care delivery system.
* Decreased agency fees by 34%.

2/90-11/93

Healthfirst Hospital, Gull, Florida
Vice President of Nursing Services
Responsible for nursing division, home health, skilled nursing
facility, emergency department, and operating room services in
250-bed unionized facility. Managed 348 full-time employees.

VICE PRESIDENT RÉSUMÉ *(continued)*

Corbin Jenkins
Page 2

Reported to CEO.
- Initiated cardiac rehabilitation program.
- Planned and supervised renovation of ED.
- Developed clinical pathways.
- Designed new employee evaluation system.
- Reduced RN vacancy rate from 22% to 2%.
- Redesigned ED classification system, saving $250,000.
- Successfully negotiated nursing contract.
- Devised multidisciplinary action plans.
- Expanded intensive care unit and trauma curriculum.

4/85-1/90

Major Hospital, Dolphin, Florida
Director of Nursing
Assisted Vice President of Nursing in administrative aspects for nursing department in 200-bed facility with 300 full-time employees. Assumed administrative call every fourth weekend and during Vice President's absence. Areas of responsibility included 138 beds, 5 operating room suites, 160 employees, 5 nurse managers, JCAHO review, budgeting, quality improvement, and risk management. Reported to Vice President of Nursing.
- Authored policies and procedures for cardiac rehabilitation program.
- Created plan for urgent care center.
- Successfully recruited three cardiologists.
- Devised housewide education program for staff and provided in-service education.
- Served as chairman of nursing quality assurance and risk management committee.
- Formulated and executed hospital-wide case management program.
- Collaborated with architects in building of three patient care units.
- Developed and coordinated start-up of new wound care center.

12/81-3/85

Gulf Shores Regional Medical Center, Santa Rosa, Florida
House Supervisor, Evenings
Responsible for hospital-wide supervision of 150-bed acute care facility on evening shift. Coordinated JCAHO activities for nursing department, resulting in maximum accreditation. Reported to Director of Nursing.

(continued)

Corbin Jenkins
Page 3

6/72-11/81

White Sands Medical Center, Beach, Florida
Nurse Manager — ICU/CCU (10/76-11/81)
Responsible for 8-bed ICU/CCU and 10-bed progressive care
unit with total of 45 full-time employees. Maintained budgeting
and conducted hiring, firing, staffing, staff education,
evaluations, and counseling. Functioned as unit resource person.
Acted as liaison for staff members, Medical Director, physicians,
ED, and admitting department. Facility is a 200-bed, county-
owned hospital. Reported to Director of Critical Care Services.
Staff Nurse — ICU/CCU (6/72-10/76)
Responsible for direct patient care on above unit. Implemented
patient and family teaching. Served as preceptor for new staff
members and taught basic ECG interpretation. Originated
assessment and charting forms. Cases included medical cardiac,
congestive heart failure, intensive postoperative, trauma,
telemetry, and respiratory patients. Reported to Nurse Manager.

5/70-5/72

Dolphin Springs Hospital, Dolphin Springs, Florida
Staff Nurse
Responsible for direct patient care on 24-bed medical/surgical
unit. Served as rotating Charge Nurse. Reported to Head Nurse.
Floated to intensive care unit when necessary. (Hospital was
76-bed, county-owned facility, which later closed.)

CERTIFICATIONS/LICENSURES

- Certified Nursing Administrator, Advanced
- CCRN
- Advanced Cardiac Life Support Provider
- Certified Professional in Health Care Quality
- RN #555-5555, Florida, expires 12/00

PROFESSIONAL AFFILIATIONS

- Florida Nurses Association, President
- American Nurses Association
- American Organization of Nurse Executives
- Florida Organization of Nurse Executives
- American Association of Critical Care Nurses
- Florida College, Adjunct Professor of Nursing
- Nurses For Life, President

VICE PRESIDENT RÉSUMÉ *(continued)*

Corbin Jenkins
Page 4

- American Red Cross Volunteer
- American College of Healthcare Executives

HONORS/AWARDS

- Sigma Theta Tau, 10/98
- Who's Who in American Nursing, 2/98
- Outstanding Alumni Award, Florida College, 5/97
- Who's Who in American Women, 1/97
- Woman of the Year, American Business Women, 1/89
- Voted Employee of the Year by White Sands Medical Center employees, 12/79
- Business & Professional Women's Young Careerist, 10/78
- Graduated Distinguished Student, Highest Honors, 6/77
- Recipient of National Nursing President's Award, 6/77
- Florida Nursing Honor Society, 6/76

PUBLICATIONS

Jenkins, Corbin, "Administrative Dilemma: Adversity in Restructuring," *Nurse Executive Journal,* 8/98

Jenkins, Corbin, "How to Manage from the Bottom Up," *Nurse Executive Journal,* 2/97

Jenkins, Corbin, "What Nurse Executives Can Learn from Their Staff," *Nurse Executive Journal,* 10/96

Jenkins, Corbin, and Scott, Sarah, "Understanding Your Managers," *CNO Today,* 8/95

PRESENTATIONS

"Daily Quality Management," Nursing Executive Conference, Los Angeles, 10/98

"The Thirty Minute Case Manager," Case Managers Conference, Tallahassee, 7/97

"How to Fail at Micromanagement," Nursing Management Conference, San Diego, 5/97

"Top Ten Ways to Burn Out," National Organization of Nurse Executives Conference, Honolulu, 10/95

"Total Quality Leadership," Quality Council, Navarre, Florida, 2/94

"The Future of Nursing," *Medicine Today* television program, Tallahassee, 11/93

"The Key is TQM," Florida Hospital Association, Tallahassee, 8/93

"Chief Nurse Executive: In or Out?" Leadership Conference, Navarre, Florida, 2/92

"Intensive Care for Managers," National Nursing Conference, Boulder, 4/89

REFERENCES
Available upon request

detail for the administrative positions, including breaking out her accomplishments into bulleted lists and, wherever possible, describing those accomplishments in concrete, measurable terms. She takes a full four pages to give the employer enough information to decide that she's the best candidate for the job; two pages just wouldn't do it.

One other detail to note on this résumé: Under the Presentations heading, the author doesn't include the state for such commonly known cities as Los Angeles and Orlando but does include it for the lesser-known city of Navarre, Florida. It's not necessary to include the state for well-known cities.

A detailed portrait

Everything you put in your résumé will lead employers to draw conclusions about you. If you were President of your nursing class, they may conclude you have a good personality and get along well with others or that you have leadership qualities. If you list 6 jobs in 3 years, they'll conclude you can't commit yourself and won't stay. If you were an Employee of the Month, they'll conclude you must be a good employee, but if you took 2 years off to travel because you needed a break, they may decide you really don't care enough about work.

Your résumé is a detailed portrait of your work history, and a good résumé is exactly what an employer needs to decide if you're the person for the job. And contrary to what some candidates think, employers actually *want* to find people to hire. Make sure your résumé provides proof to strengthen the case you're trying to make—that you can do the job.

THE COVER LETTER

A one-page cover letter should accompany every résumé. Its purpose? To spark the interest of the prospective employer, recruiter, or network contact and make them want to read your résumé. As in your résumé, use action verbs to make the letter dynamic.

Introductory paragraph

Begin by introducing yourself and stating the purpose of your letter (responding to a job listing, writing to the employer because you're targeting the company or at someone's suggestion, contacting a recruiter, and so forth) and what position you seek.

FIRST TIMER   Students, you'll also need to include:

- that you're a new graduate and the date you'll graduate
- your grade point average if it is 3.0 or higher
- any upcoming examinations you will take and the date you will take them
- the date you can begin working. ❖

Body

This is your chance to sell yourself. Tell them why you're interested in working for their company, and include specific aspects of your experience and strengths that match their needs. Choose related background and pertinent certifications and accomplishments reworded from your résumé. What qualifies you for the position? Why should they hire you? What makes you different from other candidates? Tell them why you're interested in working for them, and prove to them that you can do the job.

FIRST TIMER   Students, if you have little or no clinical experience, mention your clinical rotations. For example, highlight that your clinical rotations included working in pediatrics and on intensive care and medical-surgical units. Or you can list your patients' diagnoses, such as heart failure, appendectomy, hypertension, and so on. ❖

Closing paragraph

Reiterate your interest in the position or company here. Mention that you're enclosing your résumé and (if applicable) letters of reference. State that you'll contact them, and give them a time frame. Supply your phone number and the best time to reach you.

 FIRST TIMER   Students, make sure you mention the letters of reference you're enclosing with your résumé. ❖

Remember, keep the letter brief. Your main goal here is to catch their interest enough to read your résumé.

Sample cover letters

The following sections discuss several sample letters, including an unsolicited letter, a response to an advertisement, a letter to a recruiter, a referral letter, and an unsolicited letter from a student nurse. (See *Sample letters*, pages 73 and 75 to 78.)

Unsolicited letter

In this letter, the employer knows immediately that this candidate wants an Oncology Clinical Nurse Specialist position, that she's already filling such a position, and that she wants to work in their organization. The background she mentions is right on target for such a position. She uses the final paragraph to include contact information and when she will follow up.

Response to an advertisement

This candidate understands that employers often run advertisements for several positions simultaneously in several publications, so she mentions not only where she found the position but what position she's interested in. She then lists her qualifications and some of her pertinent accomplishments — the bullets make her accomplishments stand out. The last

UNSOLICITED LETTER

Robin O'Reilly, RN, MSN, OCN
5601 Cardinal Lane
Owensboro, Kentucky 42301
(502) 684-5555

Today's Date

Employer Name
Title
Company Name
Street Address
City, State Zip Code

Dear Mr./Ms. (Name):

My background as an Oncology Clinical Nurse Specialist may interest you. Since learning of your outstanding oncology program, I have become interested in joining your team.

Besides having 10 years' clinical hematology/oncology nursing background, including pediatric, adult, and bone marrow transplant, I also have both inpatient and outpatient experience. Last year, I was involved in the start-up of our BMT unit. My certifications include oncology, pediatric oncology, chemotherapy, ACLS, and BCLS.

I have enclosed my résumé for your review and look forward to discussing available opportunities within your organization. I will contact you the week of (month/date). If you have any questions, feel free to call me at the above number after 6:00 p.m. I look forward to speaking with you.

Sincerely,

Robin O'Reilly

RO
Enclosure

paragraph includes both day and evening numbers and states when she will contact them. One added touch: She includes a professional E-mail address at the top of her letter.

Letter to a recruiter

As illustrated in this letter, a letter to a recruiter needs to contain certain specific information, including:
- which position you seek or will consider
- your motivation for looking
- your qualifications
- your location requirements
- your salary expectations based on your current cost of living
- contact information and the best time to call.

Referral letter

The first paragraph begins by mentioning the person who referred Mariah to this employer. It also tells the employer that she just completed a Family Nurse Practitioner program and specifies when she will sit for the examination. The next paragraph covers her qualifications and certifications.

Because this candidate has such an extensive clinical background as a practicing RN in the clinical area in which she wants to work, she doesn't mention her Student Nurse Practitioner clinical experience. But, because she's seeking a position in the emergency department of a level I trauma center, she includes her emergency department rotation; in fact, any emergency, trauma, or critical care experience would be pertinent for the position she seeks. She includes two letters of reference to help offset her lack of a work history as a Family Nurse Practitioner.

(Text continues on page 79.)

ADVERTISEMENT RESPONSE LETTER

Shawnee Silvka, RN, BSN

42301 Golfview Road
Muncie, Indiana 47308

(765) 284-5555
E-mail:obnurse@source.net

Today's Date

Employer Name
Title
Company Name
Street Address
City, State Zip Code

Dear Mr./Ms. (Name):

My extensive experience is a good match for the Manager of Obstetric Services position you advertised in the *Muncie Journal-Review*.

My background includes 4 years' clinical obstetrics and 8 years' progressive management experience, encompassing high-risk labor and delivery, postpartum, and recovery. I directed the patient care of a 33-bed maternal care unit and a 30-bassinet newborn unit, supervising 65 full-time employees. My accomplishments include:

- creating and implementing an LDRP program
- implementing a unit-based Continuous Quality Improvement program
- developing "The Stork's Nest," an alternative birthing place
- achieving 100% staff certification for fetal heart monitoring.

I have enclosed my résumé and look forward to discussing this challenging opportunity within your organization. I will contact you within the next week. For additional information, you can reach me at (765) 284-3333 during the daytime or (765) 284-5555 during the evening.

Sincerely,

Shawnee Silvka

SS
Enclosure

RECRUITER LETTER

Jerry Michaels, RN, MBA

1648 Selma Boulevard
Chrisney, Indiana 47611
(812) 544-5555

Today's Date

Recruiter Name
Title
Company Name
Street Address
City, State Zip Code

Dear Mr./Ms.(Name):

My administrative experience may be of interest to your current or future clients. I seek a
Chief Nursing Officer position within a stable and progressive organization that possesses
high ethical and professional standards. My motivation for this search is to obtain increased
responsibility.

I have 18 years of progressive management and clinical operations experience. Currently, I
serve as Vice President of Nursing in a 200-bed acute care facility and manage 280 full-time
employees. I have an extensive background in work redesign, productivity enhancement, and
cost reduction. My recent efforts have focused on a hospital-wide reorganization.

I am willing to relocate, with a preference for areas east of the Mississippi River, although I
will consider other locations. My current salary is $72,000 and my lowest salary consideration
in a comparable cost-of-living area is $70,000.

I have enclosed my résumé for your review and look forward to discussing available opportunities within your client companies. I may be reached at home in the evening at the above
number or during the daytime at (812) 544-3333. However, my vacation begins on Saturday;
I will contact you on Monday the 6th when I return. Thank you for your time and
consideration.

Sincerely,

Jerry Michaels

JM
Enclosure

REFERRAL LETTER

Mariah Brandon, RN, MSN

1628 Alexander Avenue
Crawfordsville, Indiana 47933
(765) 362-4444

Today's Date

Employer Name
Title
Company Name
Street Address
City, State Zip Code

Dear Mr./Ms.(Name):

I was referred to you by Leona Norris, RN, Director of the Family
Nurse Practitioner program at the University of Indianapolis. I
recently completed my course work and will sit for the FNP
examination in October of this year. I will be available for
employment October 20th. My goal is to find a challenging FNP
position in a level I trauma center.

My RN clinical background encompasses 5 years in medical/
surgical nursing, 6 years in critical care, 4 years in pediatrics and,
most recently, 4 years in the emergency department of a level I
trauma center. Certifications including CEN, TNCC, PALS, and
CCRN have been valuable to me in the family practice area.

Enclosed are my résumé and two letters of reference. I am
interested in an opportunity with your facility and will contact you
within the next week. In the meantime, if you have any questions
you may reach me at (765) 364-5555 (daytime) or (765) 362-4444
(evenings).

Sincerely,

Mariah Brandon

MJB
Enclosures

UNSOLICITED STUDENT LETTER

Nigel Janssen

4791 Indiana Boulevard
Ottumwa, Iowa 52501
(515) 682-5555

Today's Date

Employer Name
Title
Company Name
Street Address
City, State Zip Code

Dear Mr./Ms.(Name):

After 7 years as a Nursing Assistant, I will graduate from Indian Hills Community College with an Associate of Science Degree in Nursing and a 3.9 GPA. I seek a staff RN position and would like to work within your organization. I am scheduled to sit for the NCLEX examination on (date) and will be available to begin employment on (date).

My background as a Nursing Assistant and the experience I obtained through my clinical rotations, including medical/surgical, intensive care, and progressive care, have built a firm foundation for my first nursing position. I will consider any clinical area, depending upon your needs. I am enthusiastic and dependable and have a strong commitment to quality patient care.

Please consider my résumé along with letters of reference, which I have enclosed for your review. If you need additional information, feel free to contact me at my home number listed above. Thank you for your consideration. I will be in touch with you next week to discuss further possibilities for employment.

Sincerely,

Nigel Janssen

NJ
Enclosures

Unsolicited letter from a student

FIRST TIMER   This letter lets the employer know that the candidate is a new nursing graduate and a good student. By saying he wants a staff position and not specifying any further, he shows he's flexible—a plus for a new graduate. He then tells when he'll take his NCLEX examination. ❖

The next paragraph mentions his clinical history but emphasizes his clinical rotations because he wants the employer to see him as an RN, not a Nursing Assistant. Then, although not objective, he describes a few admirable personal qualities. He concludes with contact and follow-up information.

CHOOSING YOUR REFERENCES

Finally, a few words about a tool can make or break you: your references. You'll need to choose them with great care. Most employers want references from a subordinate, a peer, and a supervisor. If you can, get a reference from an instructor or mentor; good references from doctors you've worked with also carry a lot of weight.

Make sure these people can speak about you from first-hand professional experience. Ask them if they will give you a good reference before an employer contacts them, and ask them specifically what they will say about you. If you haven't spoken with them in awhile, refresh their memories of your past relationship and your duties at that time; then update them on your current situation and your goals.

If you have any doubt about what someone will say, look for another reference; a bad reference can be your worst nightmare. (See *Know your references,* page 80.)

Letters of reference: Help for a weak résumé

A good résumé can go a long way toward convincing an employer that you're the right person for the job. But if your ré-

KNOW YOUR REFERENCES

Sally, a nurse educator, supplied a potential employer with three references. Two of them gave glowing reports of her, but the third reference didn't have one good thing to say about her. In fact, once he got started on what he thought was wrong with Sally — both professionally and personally — he couldn't seem to stop.

After several minutes of this, the hiring official's curiosity got the better of her. She finally interrupted and asked, "Why did you agree to be a reference for Sally? Didn't she know how you felt about her?" He replied, "I did it because Sally asked me to."

Sally's mistake? She'd neglected to ask her references what they'd actually say about her.

sumé is weak — maybe because you lack experience or changed jobs frequently — it won't make it through the first cut on its own. In that case, you may want to submit letters of reference with the résumé. If you do, make sure all the people who write letters for you:

- know they may be contacted
- will write outstanding letters of reference (mediocre ones won't do)
- will keep your job search in strictest confidence if you're currently employed.

The right tools will present you in the best professional manner. Now that you have a good résumé in hand and know how to write an appropriate cover letter and choose the best references, you're ready to plan your strategy, handle interviews with confidence — and get the offer you want.

4

THE PLAN

You've completed your assessment. You know what you want in a position and where you will or won't go geographically. Your résumé and cover letters present a professional first impression to prospective employers.

But how do you get the word out that you're in the market for a new position? How do you learn about opportunities that are right for you? Should you use a recruiter? What if you're a student? This chapter can help you answer these questions and develop a marketing plan that's right for you.

NETWORKING

One of the most crucial aspects of planning—and maybe your best bet for hearing about the position you want—is to develop a strong professional network. In fact, whether you're actively job seeking or not, you should always maintain and expand your network. If you don't, you'll be faced with the daunting task of rebuilding your network every time you start a new job search; having a network in place when you need it can literally cut off months of a job search.

Picture it this way: When you start out, your network is like a young tree just beginning to put out branches. Over time, with care and nurturing, these branches begin to grow and spread, forming an ever-expanding network. Soon your tree is putting out even more branches and thousand of telescoping twigs. So it goes with a carefully planned network. As you can see, a strong network gives you nearly limitless potential that you could never match on your own.

Building your network

Tailor your networking plan to fit your situation. If you're employed and don't want word to get out at work that you're looking, you'll have to be careful who you tell, which makes networking more difficult. But if you're a student or unemployed, the sky is the limit! The more contacts you make, the better your chances are of finding the right position. Here's what you need to do:

- Start by brainstorming. Include everyone you know; omit no one. List friends, family members, business contacts, peers, fellow committee members, your boss, your boss's boss, subordinates, people from church, parents of your children's friends, school friends, professors, contacts at community organizations, members of professional organizations—everyone. Any one of them could lead to the right job.
- Make up business cards. Carry them with you, and give or send one to each person you contact.
- Join national and state professional associations, and attend conferences. Many state organizations have local quarterly chapter meetings (see the appendix Nursing Resources).
- Go to job fairs. Take your business cards and copies of your résumé with you.
- Contact recruiters who specialize in nursing. They can answer questions about the market on a national scale.
- If you've been let go for any reason, contact your facility's human resources department. People there may know of openings in another facility. Also, ask if the department works with an outplacement service. Such services, usu-

ally paid for by the facility that laid off the employee, can help in your job search. They offer counseling to help you cope with the loss of your job, help you prepare a résumé and cover letters, aid in networking, and more.

 FIRST TIMER   If you're a student, make sure you know everyone in your class by name and how to reach them. Prepare an address book and make notes about other students; carry it with you. By graduation, you should have useful data about every student, including address and area of specialty. Over time, these future professionals will spread throughout the country, giving you contacts nationwide.

- Talk with your nursing instructors about creating a bulletin board that students can use to post job opportunities. For instance, you might post information about a position that you interviewed for but that wasn't right for you; it might be the right fit for another student. Postings should include contact information, responsibilities, and requirements.

- Check with your school's career center. Most are quite helpful in finding leads. ❖

Organization is the key to a good network. Document (sound familiar?) names and any follow-up that occurred, keeping good records. And remember to update your network constantly, not just when you're job searching.

ADVERTISEMENTS

Don't overlook the job listings in professional journals and newspapers; you may find your next position there. Look in publications that advertise positions in the locations where you'd like to live. Don't just look in one or two sources; get your hands on as many publications as you can, including local newspapers.

The right response

Read each ad carefully, noting what qualifications the employer requires. If you have those qualities, skills, and experience and want to learn more about the position, write your response letter accordingly. Use the same terms used in the ad to describe your qualifications, and follow the instructions carefully.

If you're answering an ad that doesn't list a contact person, address the letter, "Dear Sir or Madam." If at all possible, get the contact person's name and title, and submit your cover letter and résumé directly to that person. (See *Get the right name.*) Double-check the address; if you're sending your letter directly to the hiring official, you may have more

INSIDE TRACK

GET THE RIGHT NAME

Addressing your cover letter to the right person increases your chances of getting your résumé reviewed. If nothing else, it shows you have initiative.

One way to find the name you need is to call the facility directly. Say to the operator, "I want to send a communication to the Director of Human Resources, but I don't know the person's name. Do you know who that would be?" The operator will usually have that information. If not, ask to be transferred to the appropriate department, and ask your question again.

When you have the name, double-check that you're spelling it correctly, even if you think you already are. Many names, such as Linda/Lynda, Mark/Marc, Judy/Judi, or Smith/Smyth, can lead to misspellings. If the person has a unisex name, such as Corbin, Morgan, Chris, or Sidney, also ask whether you should use *Ms.* or *Mr.* to avoid an unwitting error.

success if you send it to the main hospital address instead of the human resources post office box listed in the ad.

Your best option is to send two responses: one to human resources and one to the department with the opening. The department head may want to consider you for other positions—maybe for a new position she's developing or as a replacement for an employee she's thinking of letting go or who may want a change. The human resources contact usually isn't aware of a position until it's officially available.

Checking older sources

Check older advertisements, too; many nursing positions remain open for some time. Look through older nursing journals, and call to see if promising positions are still open. Many won't be, but a surprising number will be. The advantage? You'll have missed the first wave of applicants and, by now, the employer will be thrilled to get your résumé.

THE INTERNET

One of the newest sources for career information, the Internet is also one of the most powerful—and its importance will only increase. The Internet offers a wealth of information on professional organizations, nursing positions and recruiters, bulletin boards, hospitals, publications, and nationwide classified advertisements (for Internet listings, see the appendix Nursing Resources).

Here's just one example of how the Internet can help you in your search: Say you're a family nurse practitioner looking for a position in a certain town. You can use the Internet to get a list of the names, addresses, and phone numbers of all the family practice doctors in that area. You can then print it and send your résumé and cover letter directly to each doctor.

So if you don't have a computer, buy one; if you can't buy one, get access to one. Once you have a computer, hook up with a commercial carrier, such as America Online, CompuServe, or Microsoft Network, and get an E-mail address. To avoid long-distance charges, you can instead use a local access number or local carrier; most computer stores can give you recommendations.

PROFESSIONAL RECRUITERS

Another potentially important part of your networking plan is the professional recruiter, often called a headhunter. Recruiters work in several ways: Contingency recruiters only get paid when they fill a job or find you a position, so they'll want to place you as quickly as possible. Retained search firms receive a fee to fill a specific position and won't be interested in working with you unless your background fits a position they want to fill. Some firms handle both contingency and retained search assignments. Many firms are part of an affiliate network; firms in such a network allow each other access to their openings or candidates or both.

Keep in mind that recruiters get paid for getting results, so they'll devote their time to candidates they feel they can place. If you're such a candidate, a recruiter can help you enormously by taking the time to market your background to potential employers.

What makes you a good candidate?

A recruiter will consider you a Most Placeable Candidate if you:

- already have experience doing the kind of job you're seeking
- have appropriate salary expectations

- have a history of staying with a job (although job-hopping doesn't make the recruiter's task impossible, just more difficult)
- are willing and able to relocate (looking in only one location narrows your options tremendously)
- know what you want (this is where your blueprint comes in)
- are serious about changing jobs, not just curious
- work with one or two main recruiters, not several; more is not always better (if you're working with lots of recruiters, any one recruiter's odds for placing you go down; this lessens the recruiter's incentive to spend a lot of time trying to place you—which in turn decreases your chances of getting a job offer)
- make yourself easy to work with; you'll damage your chances with a recruiter if you're verbally abusive, don't take direction well, act defensively, or aren't up front with the recruiter.

What a recruiter can do for you

A good recruiter can usually offer you some important advantages. For instance, recruiters who work specifically in nursing know the market. Because they routinely interact with nurses and hiring officials, they know which facilities are downsizing and closing units and which are opening new units. In other words, they network in your market all day, every day—something you don't have time to do. They can watch the market on your behalf and screen positions against your background while you work or go to school. A recruiter can:

- speak to an employer about your background, calling attention to strengths in your résumé that might have been overlooked, or convince a hiring official to take another look at a résumé she would otherwise reject

- ask questions of an employer that you may feel uncomfortable asking or that you shouldn't ask
- clear up misunderstandings resulting from poor communication during an interview
- explain frequent job changes (if they were for valid reasons) when you wouldn't have gotten the chance
- help during the interview process, preparing you for telephone and on-site interviews and guiding you through salary negotiations.

How do you choose?

If you decide to use recruiters, start by doing your research. Find reputable firms that handle your discipline. Check professional journals and the Internet, network at conferences, and ask nursing instructors, mentors, and peers. Most recruiters work nationwide, so don't let location be a factor in your choice; many also have toll-free numbers. Interview recruiters on the phone to help determine which ones you feel comfortable working with.

Before making any decisions about recruiting firms, find out the answers to these questions:

- Do they specialize in nursing?
- Are they members of the National Association of Personnel Services? This national organization requires each member to subscribe to and endorse the Standards of Ethical Practices as a condition of membership.
- Do they understand your discipline or, better yet, have nurses on staff?
- Do they ask the right questions and enough questions?
- Do they take the time to speak with you and answer questions, even if they don't think they can place you? Maybe you're a student looking for guidance and won't graduate for a few years. Firms that take the time to answer your

questions now are the ones to contact when you're in the market for a new job.

- Are the recruiters Certified Personnel Consultants? Personnel consultants who've been in the industry at least 2 years can take a national examination to receive certification in their field. Administered by the National Association of Personnel Services, the examination consists of legal questions, business situations, and standards of practice. To remain certified, recruiters must also take continuing education units.
- Will they let you check their references?
- Do they charge their candidates? You shouldn't have to pay a fee for their services.
- Will they get your permission before sending out your résumé? You should know where your résumé has been sent.

Working well with recruiters

Once you've chosen a main recruiting firm to work with— and keep in mind that choosing a firm doesn't exclude you from working with other recruiters—take the time and effort to make the relationship work. Be persistent and follow up. Recruiters work with thousands of candidates, some of whom aren't seriously in the job market! When you're persistent, you let recruiters know they're not wasting their time on you. Also, treat recruiters with respect—and honesty. (See *Lying never pays,* page 90.) If you do, you'll receive the same treatment in return. Remember, the recruiter is your link to the employer.

You should also keep excellent records. Use a notebook to keep a record of recruiter contacts. Write down where a recruiter sends your résumé—including the date, the name of the facility, and its location—the name and company of the recruiter, any action taken, and follow-up; when you're

LYING NEVER PAYS

Donna, a Director of Surgical Services, used a recruiting firm to help her find a position in a new location. She accepted an offer but said she needed 3 months before starting. Although not thrilled, the employer agreed to wait.

A week before her start date, Donna called the employer and said she'd changed her mind and didn't want to relocate. Both the employer and the recruiter had spoken with her several times during the 3 months, and she'd never mentioned the possibility of not relocating. The employer was furious — not only with Donna but also with the recruiter. The employer had wasted months on this candidate and now had to begin a new search. To make matters worse, the second-choice candidate had already taken another position.

A few months later, the recruiter found out that Donna had accepted another position and had, in fact, relocated. Shortly after that, she asked that same recruiter to help her find another position. Not surprisingly, the recruiter was not interested in representing her.

well into your search, it's easy to start confusing hospitals with similar names.

Also, keep a record of any contacts you make yourself. For instance, if you reply to an advertisement yourself or if you have your own lead on a job and send in a résumé, record the date, the name of the facility and its location, the position, the contact person, and the phone and fax numbers. Check back periodically with the contact person.

Keep in mind that once you've applied on your own, an employer won't work with a recruiter on your behalf. And when you work with a recruiter for a specific position, you shouldn't contact the employer unless the recruiter advises you to do so.

When not to use a recruiter

In some cases, using a recruiter may not be your best option. For instance, if you're switching from one area of expertise to another, a recruiter would have a tough time placing you. Why? Because employers pay recruiters large fees to find people who can hit the ground running. Employers can run advertisements themselves to find inexperienced candidates who want to try new areas.

You should also not use recruiters if you can only work in a specific location and have already saturated that area with your résumé and cover letter. Once you've submitted a résumé, a recruiter can't work with that employer on your behalf.

Finally, if you're a new RN who has just completed a nurse practitioner bridge program, you'll do better on your own. Most employers want an employee who has a minimum of 4 years experience in the specialty area as an RN before becoming a nurse practitioner.

THE RIGHT PLAN

Planning is hard work. You'll have to network constantly, comb through advertisements, check out job resources on the Internet, choose whether or not to use recruiters, and maintain detailed records. But the right plan can help you find what employers and jobs that are out there — and, more importantly, let the right employer find you.

5

THE INTERVIEWS

As you reach the interview stage, keep in mind that the employer wants to hire the most qualified candidate. Bringing aboard a new employee is costly—interview and relocation expenses, training costs, signing bonuses, and recruiter's fees add up— so the hiring official wants to make the best decision. When she brings you in for an interview, she'll be looking for reasons to hire you. And it's *your* responsibility to give her the information she needs to offer you the job.

WHAT THE EMPLOYER NEEDS TO KNOW

During the interview process, you must bring out certain key points (provided they're true, of course). First and foremost, you must convince the employer that *you can do the job*. This is your mission, and it's critical. If you don't give the interviewer the evidence she needs to come to that conclusion, nothing else you do will matter. You won't get the job. Period.

Next, make sure the interviewer knows that y*ou want to live in that location*. The employer wants employees who want to become part of the local community. If you already live locally and don't want to relocate, tell the interviewer that you want to stay put. You'll have an advantage in this situation because you'll already know and like the area. Plus, the employer will have lower costs for interviews and no cost for relocation; if you at least live in the state, your relocation costs will be lower. If you don't live nearby, give the interviewer convincing reasons why you would want to move to the new location. Maybe the new job would put you closer to your extended family, or maybe you were originally from that area and want to move back.

You'll also need to make it clear that *you seek longevity and plan to stay put*. Of course, no one knows what the future will bring, but it's not to your or the employer's advantage to change jobs frequently. If you've been at your current position for several years, mention that; it shows the employer that you aren't a job-hopper.

Convince the interviewer that *you share the company's interests* and that your philosophy, management style, and goals are in line with the employer's. And make sure she knows that *you're committed to the job*. Give the interviewer examples, maybe from your current job, of how motivated and enthusiastic you are.

Finally, the employer *must* know that *you want the job*. The interviewer can't read your mind. Tell her, point-blank, that you want this job. If you can't get these key points across, you're wasting the employer's time—and your own.

FIRST CONTACT

Once a hiring official thinks you warrant a closer look, she'll contact you. She may want to interview you first on the telephone and call to schedule a mutually agreeable time. If so, allow at least an hour of uninterrupted time for the interview and be ready about 15 minutes before the hiring official is due to call. If you must take the call at another number, make sure you give the correct number. A scheduled interview gives you a chance to prepare.

Unfortunately, the hiring official—especially if a doctor— may call without warning and expect to conduct an on-the-spot interview. (You'll probably be in the middle of painting your dining room or having your child's birthday party when this happens!) If you receive such a call, ask politely if you could reschedule and choose a mutually convenient time. You must be mentally prepared for a telephone interview to be successful.

The hiring official may instead decide to skip the telephone interview and call to schedule an on-site interview. This is more likely if you live locally or relatively close by but can sometimes happen even if you live out of state. Bypassing the telephone interview makes the whole process proceed more quickly.

If the hiring official does choose to schedule a phone interview first, make sure you double-check the time for the call, especially if you're in a different time zone than the employer. And don't rely on your phone book's map of time zones because some areas of the country don't follow daylight savings time.

As mentioned in chapter 3, The Tools, make sure you have a professional phone message on your answering machine or voice mail. Teach children and other family members to answer the phone properly. Check your messages frequently during the day, schedule permitting, and return those messages promptly. If you get the employer's voice mail when you call, leave a detailed message that includes your name, the reason for your call, your number, and the best time to reach you. Then repeat your name and number at the end of the message. Speak clearly and slowly enough for someone hearing the message to have a chance to write it down accurately.

THE TELEPHONE INTERVIEW

The telephone interview is a chance for both sides to do some selling and get a little information about each other. The employer wants to find out if it's worth the time and expense to interview you in person. You want to find out if you're interested in learning more about the position—maybe see the unit and facility; meet with staff members, peers, and management; and check out the community if the position calls for you to relocate. But your main goal is to convince the employer to invite you for an on-site interview.

Before the phone interview

The telephone interview may be your first direct contact with the employer, so you'll need to prepare for the call:

- If possible, schedule the interview for when you'll be at your best—not late afternoon or evening if you're a morning person, for instance. If you're tired, it may come across as disinterest or a lack of energy.
- If you're taking the call at home, tell every member of your family to stay off the phone until you give them the "all clear." (See *Keep the line open,* page 96.)
- Take the call in a private area where you won't be interrupted. If an emergency arises, ask the interviewer if you can reschedule.
- Make sure you'll be out of earshot of children, barking dogs, television, radio, dishwasher, and any other noises.
- If you find out you won't be able to take the call at the scheduled time, immediately call and tell the employer.
- The interviewer will have a copy of your résumé in front of her; so should you. Review its contents before the call. It will help you keep dates straight and answer specific questions about each position. If you're not familiar with

KEEP THE LINE OPEN

Debbie, an obstetrics manager, had a telephone interview scheduled for 7 p.m. at her home, but her phone never rang. The next morning, Debbie called the recruiter and told her she'd waited over 2 hours for a call that never came. She told her that the employer had acted unprofessionally and said in no uncertain terms that she wasn't sure if she wanted to work for someone like that.

But in talking with the irate employer, the recruiter learned that she *had* tried to call—for over an hour and a half. As it turned out, Debbie's teenage daughter had been on the phone upstairs in her room all evening, so the employer had gotten nothing but a busy signal.

what's on your résumé, the interviewer will have doubts about you, and you won't hear from her again.

- Be prepared to answer questions about short-term positions and gaps in employment that appear on your résumé and to explain why you're looking for a position. Remain positive; don't get defensive.
- Know your strengths and weaknesses beforehand, and be ready to explain what you've done to work on those weaknesses.

During the phone interview

These tips can help you make the right impression:

- Don't drink, eat, smoke, chew gum, or tap a pencil during the interview.
- Avoid interruptions: Don't answer call waiting if any calls come in during the interview, and don't answer the door.
- Take notes during the interview. They can help enormously in preparing for an on-site interview.

- Be enthusiastic, and make sure your interest comes across not only in your words but also in your voice. Neither you nor the employer will have the benefit of reading body language and facial expressions.
- Be yourself, and speak in your typical conversational manner. Try to relax, but remember, a little stress is normal and may even help keep you alert.
- If you're a hiring official and interviewing for a new position, resist the temptation to take over the interview and ask all the questions (even though it's a natural tendency!).
- If you've left a position, explain as positively as possible why you left, and always mention what you learned while you were there.
- Never, under any circumstance, say anything negative about a former or current employer, no matter what happened.
- If the interviewer asks if you've done something and you have, don't just answer yes. Give an example; it helps her to picture you doing the job.
- Don't bring up salary or benefits. Interviewers rarely discuss such subjects during a phone interview. You'll also need more information before you can arrive at your own bottom line, including what the position encompasses and the relative cost of living. Plus, you don't want to be the one to come up with the salary figure. If you do, it becomes *their* decision; if they come up with the figure, it's *your* decision.
- As the interview progresses and you discover what the employer needs, give the interviewer examples from your background that show you can meet those needs.
- Ask two or three questions of your own that you've prepared beforehand. For instance, you might ask what the interviewer sees the person who takes this job doing in the first 6 months. You could also ask what the facility's

mission statement is and whether the facility has gone through a reorganization. Remember, the questions you ask help reveal your priorities to the interviewer. Having no questions shows a lack of interest.

- Be ready with a couple of dates when you could meet for an interview, in case they ask. If you don't live near the company, plan extra time for travel the day before the interview so that you can stay nearby overnight if necessary; many interviews begin first thing in the morning. If you live nearby, you won't need to spend the night.

- At the end of the interview, if you're still interested in learning more about the position and going on-site, let the interviewer know. Ask if she can send you a recruitment packet, a job description, and an application that you can complete before the interview.

After the phone interview

Unless you learned something about the position during the phone interview that you absolutely can't live with, you owe it to yourself to go in for an on-site interview. If you're going to make an informed decision, you need to learn all of the details about the position; visit the facility; meet your potential supervisor, peers, subordinates; and tour the community. If you don't go, you'll never really know what the opportunity could mean to your career.

THE ON-SITE INTERVIEW

An employer who invites you for an on-site interview is considering you very seriously for the position. Such interviews can cost the employer considerable time and money, even for a local candidate; if the employer must fly you in, the costs are even higher. So, although coming in for an interview doesn't commit you to accepting an offer, it does mean you'll come into the interview with an open mind and honestly consider the position. If you already *know* you won't take the position or move to that location, don't go. But if you're seriously interested, it's time to prepare to meet your potential employer face to face.

Keep your goals in mind when preparing for the interview. You want to get the job offer, of course. But you also want to find out if the position matches your personal blueprint (see chapter 2, The Assessments). The on-site interview is a chance to do both.

Gather your information

You'll need to be organized and plan carefully to ensure a successful interview with no unpleasant surprises. Start by completing an interview data sheet so that you have all the information you need at your fingertips. (See *Interview data,* page 100.)

Doing your homework

You may have asked for a recruitment packet, job description, and application during the phone interview. Now go to the library and research the facility yourself. What type of facility is it? Who owns it? How many beds does it have? What services does it provide? The American Hospital Association Guide should give you most of this information. If you may relocate, contact the new location's chamber of commerce and ask for a newcomer's packet. You can use all of this information to help you prepare for the interview.

Prepare for the questions

A crucial part of your preparation is thinking about the questions you'll be asked and those you will ask the interviewer. Start by recognizing that you and the interviewer have different backgrounds and life experiences and thus different

INTERVIEW DATA

INTERVIEWER AND TITLE:

PHONE NUMBER: FAX NUMBER:

FACILITY NAME:

FACILITY ADDRESS:

CITY, STATE, AND ZIP CODE:

AFTER-HOURS CONTACT AND PHONE NUMBER:

POSITION TITLE:

INTERVIEWS SCHEDULED:

A.M./P.M.:   TIME ZONE:

DAY: DATE:

DEPARTMENT AND LOCATION:

AIRLINE INFORMATION:

HOTEL:

HOTEL PHONE AND CONFIRMATION NUMBERS:

TRANSPORTATION:

PARKING:

REMARKS:

DIRECTIONS:

priorities. Each interviewer will have a different set of questions that reflect what is important to her. You'll need to listen carefully to determine how to respond and what accomplishments, skills, and experiences you should highlight. And you'll need to determine what kinds of questions you should ask of the employer. Don't forget your mission: to give the interviewer evidence that you can do job.

Questions the employer might ask

Although the specific questions you'll face may vary, some types of questions tend to occur more often than others. Knowing beforehand what those questions are and how to answer them can help make your interviews more successful. (See *Handling the fundamental questions,* pages 102 and 103.)

You might also want to think about how you would respond to the following:

- Describe your typical day. What's your energy level?
- Why did you choose this vocation?
- When you leave your current position, what three things might your boss say about you? Your coworkers? Your staff?
- What did you like best about your favorite boss? What did you like least about your worst boss? (Answer these questions with caution.)
- In which previous position do you think you accomplished the most?
- What three things did you do to make progress in your department?
- What do you like most about your clinical area? What do you like least?
- What changes do you think need to be made in our facility?

Questions you might ask

You should get a chance to ask questions, too. It helps to prepare some carefully thought out questions before the interview. Look over the following list to see which might work for you.

- How long has the position been open?
- Why is it open?
- Could I see a copy of the job description?

HANDLING THE FUNDAMENTAL QUESTIONS

No matter who you interview with, you'll face fundamental questions about yourself, your qualifications, and your reasons for changing jobs. Below you'll find some of those questions, along with suggestions on how to prepare your answers.

Question: Why do you want to make a job change?
How to answer: If you are employed and looking to change jobs, mention the positive points about the new position. Explain what sparked your interest—maybe the increase in challenge and responsibility, better hours, a chance to work closer to home, or a chance for advancement that you don't have in your current job.

Question: Why did you leave your last position?
How to answer: Give an objective reason why you left, and mention three things you learned while you were at your last job. Keep your answer positive, even if it's a challenge to do so.

Question: Could you tell me something about yourself?
How to answer: Narrow the focus of this question by asking the interviewer where she'd like you to begin, and keep your answer work related.

Question: What have you learned about our company, and why would you like to work for us?
How to answer: Draw on the research that you did on the company before the interview to give the interviewer a well-informed answer.

Question: How do you differ from other candidates, and why should I hire you?
How to answer: Know your accomplishments, experience, and skills so that you can tell the interviewer what you have to offer. You must know

HANDLING THE FUNDAMENTAL QUESTIONS *(continued)*

the answer to this question; if you can't tell the interviewer why she should hire you, stay at home.

Question: What are your strengths and your weaknesses?
How to answer: Start by telling the interviewer your strengths, with examples. But be ready to discuss your weaknesses (everyone has a weakness), along with what you're doing to correct those weaknesses.

Question: How do you handle yourself during stressful situations?
How to answer: Use examples to demonstrate how you react to and cope with stressful situations.

Question: Are you willing to relocate? Why would you want to move here?
How to answer: The personal and professional assessment you did earlier will supply you with a ready answer for this question. Community information gathered from the local newspaper and chamber of commerce can also help.

Question: Have you ever started a unit, been involved in a renovation, or taken part in any similar major change?
How to answer: Don't just say yes: Give concrete examples from your experience.

Question: What goals have you set for yourself?
How to answer: Make sure you have some! If you aim at nothing, you'll probably hit it.

- What kind of orientation program do you have?
- How do you envision this position?
- What do you see the person who takes this position doing in the first 6 months?

- What is the facility's philosophy?
- Does the facility have plans for future growth?
- Has the facility recently reorganized?
- Do you have a copy of the organizational chart?
- How many beds are on the unit?
- What specific types of patients are on this unit?
- What's the average census on the unit?
- Does this unit run smoothly?
- What challenges might the person who takes this position face?
- Is the staff fairly new or more seasoned? Is it stable?
- What is the nurse-patient ratio?

Prepare for the interview

Now that you've prepared for the questions that may arise during the interview and planned the questions you'll ask, it's time to focus on the logistics of preparing for the interview itself.

 ON THE MOVE   If you must travel for the interview, you'll need to take a few extra steps to prepare:

- If you'll be flying, carry a picture identification with you. You may want to ask your travel agent or an airline representative what you'll need because some carriers require two forms of identification.
- Get a confirmation number when making a hotel reservation, and keep that number with you.
- Save all receipts and jot down what each one was for. When you submit these receipts for reimbursement, keep a copy for your records.
- If you're scheduled to arrive on a weekend or holiday or after business hours, have the contact person's home number with you in case a problem arises.
- If you need to rent a car, have a valid driver's license and a major credit card with you, and make sure you meet the

rental company's age requirements. You may want to call ahead to ask about their requirements and to confirm your car reservation.

- Request an itinerary so you'll know your schedule. It will also have the titles and correctly spelled names of everyone you'll be meeting with — useful for writing follow-up letters.

- You may want to ask the employer to recommend a realtor to give you a tour of the area. ❖

Making a good impression

Some planning before the interview can help you make the best impression:

- Although not always possible, try to get a good night's sleep the night before the interview. Don't try to work extra hours the day before to get the time off that you need; that can backfire.

- Wear business attire and polished shoes. Choose dark colors and conservative jewelry; this isn't the time to make a fashion statement. Avoid heavy perfume or cologne and heavy makeup, wear deodorant, and follow proper oral hygiene. Don't put off that hair cut until after the interview, and make sure your nails are well groomed. You want to be remembered for your excellent qualifications, not your poor appearance.

- Use an attaché or portfolio to carry several clean copies of your résumé, a completed application (if you have one), paper, and any brochures, policies and procedures manuals, or programs you developed. Have a nice pen handy, not one you picked up at the airport that says "Barney's Bar and Grill" on it; the little things people notice about you can make a difference.

- Plan to arrive at the interview 15 minutes early; you must not arrive late. Stop by and use the rest room when you arrive, and take the time to check your appearance and run warm water over your hands if they're ice-cold from nervousness. Keep your caffeine intake to its normal level.

- Go to the first destination listed on your interview data sheet, introduce yourself, and explain why you're there. Treat every person you meet with respect, friendliness, and courtesy. Treating anyone — receptionists, secretaries, or human resource representatives — with rudeness may hurt your chances of getting the job.

Filling out the application

If you haven't yet filled out an employment application and you receive one, read through the directions first. Fill out the application completely. If a question doesn't apply to you, write "N/A" (not applicable). Don't lie on the application; it's grounds for termination. Have your social security and nursing license numbers with you. If the application has a line for salary expectations, write down something such as "I will consider a fair offer." (The salary is just a piece of the whole package.) Under the past and current employment section, don't write "see résumé" (this is a pet peeve of employers); list each previous and current employer completely, using the information from your résumé. Print neatly, and proofread the whole application after you're finished.

Make the interview a success

You want to do everything in your power to make sure the employer offers you the job. These tips can guide you through the interview itself:

- Greet the employer by name, and shake hands firmly. Use the interviewer's name during the interview.
- Make eye contact, but don't stare.
- Don't sit until offered a chair. Maintain good posture at all times, and be alert; your body language speaks volumes.

SHOW THEM THE REAL YOU

Derick, an enthusiastic and qualified medical/surgical educator, couldn't wait until his on-site interview. The position the recruiter had found for him was just what he was looking for and a perfect match for his background. The prospective employer also liked Derick's experience and thought he had a lot to offer, so they flew him in for a full day of interviews.

After the interview, the recruiter couldn't believe the feedback she got from the employer. "Derick seemed uninterested and had no enthusiasm. We're no longer interested in him," the hiring official told her. The recruiter almost thought they were talking about another person, not the Derick she knew. When the recruiter spoke with Derick, he was still very interested in the position, but he told her that he'd had an allergy attack and had taken an allergy pill before the interview. "It was pretty bad," he said. "I could hardly keep my eyes open."

Unfortunately, the employer wasn't interested in spending another $800 to bring him back for a second chance.

- Don't keep looking at your watch.
- Show enthusiasm, and let the interviewer know you're glad to be there. Employers need to see that you're excited about the possibility of working for them. (See *Show them the real you.*)
- Ask permission to take notes; then jot down any pertinent information. You can use your notes later to help you process everything you heard. Taking notes also shows your interest, gives you something to do with your hands, and helps decrease your stress.
- Sometimes an interviewer can start with a question such as, "Why don't you tell me something about yourself?" Such an open-ended question can lead to disastrous re-

sults. Tell the interviewer you'd be happy to, and ask where she'd like you to start. This lets her focus in on what she wants to know. Stick to work-related information in your answer.

- Listen carefully to the questions, and don't interrupt. Take a moment before answering if you need to. If you don't know the answer to a question, don't make up something; just tell the interviewer you don't know. If the interviewer asks if you've done something and you have, give an example to help her picture you doing the job.

 FIRST TIMER   If you're a graduate applying for your first job, don't apologize for your shortcomings. The interviewer already knows you're just starting out. Instead, let her know you're eager to learn and will put in the extra time and effort needed. ❖

- Have ready a list of your accomplishments. Then, listen to what the interviewer says and the questions she asks. As you learn about the facility's needs, interject your accomplishments and experiences accordingly. For instance, if the facility plans on remodeling the emergency department and you've been through that, let the interviewer know. Matching the employer's needs to your background will put you ahead of the pack.

- Demonstrate that you would be a dedicated worker.

- Don't talk about controversial subjects, such as religion and politics; you could end up in a disagreement. And never discuss personal problems.

- Don't lie to the interviewer. Be ready to answer honestly questions about gaps in your job history or frequent job changes, and keep a positive attitude.

- Never make negative comments about your current or former employers, no matter how much you feel they deserve it. Even if you hit it off with the interviewer, don't get too comfortable and start talking about how unfair your last boss was. It's a fatal move.

- Don't complain, period. If your flight was late or your hotel room was terrible, keep it to yourself or you won't leave a favorable impression. Your focus should be on the job and what you can do for the employer.

- Don't bring up benefits, paid time off, bonuses, retirement, or anything like that. You can get information about such things later from human resources.

- If you're taken out to lunch or dinner, don't smoke or drink, even if the interviewer urges you to do so. You may feel like you're done and it's time to relax but if you're still with the interviewer, the interview isn't really finished. *You must remain on your best behavior.*

- If the interviewer asks you what salary you want, tell her you'll consider a fair offer. If she presses further, tell her you'll need more information to arrive at a specific figure — for instance, a cost-of-living comparison if you'll have to relocate. It's not a good idea for you to come up with a number. A figure that's too high puts you out of contention; one that's too low will cost you money. You're not likely to be right on target. Let the employer start with a figure and work from there.

 FIRST TIMER   Unfortunately, you won't have much bargaining power if you're a new graduate. With little or no experience, you'll probably be on the low end of the wage scale. But there may be some room for negotiation, so if you're asked what you need, say that you'll consider a fair offer. ❖

- Remember to ask some of the questions you've prepared for the interview. You can interject your questions at appropriate times during the interview. For instance, you might ask about the facility's short- and long-range objectives, its growth plans, the management philosophy, and the area you could contribute most effectively. The questions you ask will tell the employer about your priorities.

- Do your best throughout the interview, even if you decide you're not interested shortly after the interview begins. Your goal is still to get the job offer. Then the decision is yours, not theirs. If you give up on the interview partway through and then change your mind and decide you want the job, it will be too late.

- At the end of each interview, ask for a business card so that you'll have correct names and titles for follow-up letters.

10 ways to lose the job

Now that you know how to handle yourself in an interview so that you get the job, look over these ways other candidates have inadvertently made sure they didn't get the job:

1. Tell the interviewer how unfair your last boss was. This will get her on your side.

2. Arrive a few minutes late. You hate to wait; it makes you nervous. Besides, you don't want them to think you're too anxious.

3. Try to gather as much information during the interview as possible by reading papers or files on the interviewer's desk. Move things on the desk so you can get a better look.

4. Let the interviewer know how your day is going. Complain about your headache, not having enough coffee, the way you were treated at the airport, and how grueling your interview schedule is. This will leave a lasting impression.

5. Don't bother to prepare. You've interviewed lots of times; plus, you conduct interviews yourself. Piece of cake!

6. Have an attitude that says, "What can you do for me?" Let the interviewer know how much money you must have, what benefits you require, and when you already have your vacation scheduled. They can take it or leave it. You're worth it.

7. When asked about future goals, tell them you don't have any.

8. Take your potential new boss out for drinks after the interview. You two really hit it off and you know you've got the job in the bag. Celebrate!

9. Don't ask questions. No need to. Either you already know everything or you don't know enough to ask questions.

10. Tell the interviewer your entire family history in great detail, including the highlights of your messy divorce.

Wrap up the interview gracefully

When you get to the end of your interview, make sure you end on the best note possible. Thank the hiring official for her time, and tell her how much you enjoyed meeting everyone. Make some positive comments; maybe the unit was newly renovated and looked very impressive, for instance. If you want the position and can do the job, tell the hiring official point blank; this isn't the time to be shy. Then, ask when you might be hearing from her.

It isn't normal practice to offer a candidate the job at the interview, but it does occasionally happen. Most employers will want to get feedback from everyone you've interviewed with or they may have other candidates to interview before making a final decision. But if you receive an offer with an acceptable salary and you know you want the job, accept it. If you need some time—to discuss the offer with your family, decide if the offer is fair, or check out the area—ask if you can have a couple of days to get back to the employer.

Send out follow-up letters quickly

Within 48 hours of returning home, send follow-up letters to the main interviewers—usually the person to whom you would be reporting, peers you interviewed with, and the human resources representative. Make sure you address each of them by name. Don't use your present employer's letterhead; instead, use good quality, plain white or cream-colored, 24-lb stationery. Thank each person for their hospitality and the chance to interview with them; if you want the position, say so again in your letter. Reiterate the qualifications and strengths you have that fit the employer's needs (you should know those needs well by now). Mention highlights of the interview and things that impressed you. Triple-check these letters for errors. If you fail to get the letters out within 48 hours, send them by overnight delivery. (See *Sample follow-up letter.*)

If you arrive home and decide you definitely won't consider the position, no matter what the offer, don't make the facility come up with an offer just to see what you would have gotten. The work in putting a package together for a candidate can be immense. A hiring official may have to pull a few strings to get a better package for a strong candidate. It's not professional to put someone through this if you know you're going to turn down the offer.

Instead, send a letter to the person who extended the offer and thank her for her hospitality and the opportunity to interview at the facility. Let the employer know that you don't feel the position would be a good fit for you at this time. (Don't say that you don't like the facility, the management team was rude, or it would take you a lifetime to get that place in shape.) If the company feels you're not a good match for the position, the hiring official should afford you the same courtesy, either by telephone or mail.

SAMPLE FOLLOW-UP LETTER

Alexis Bright
2322 Miramar Boulevard
Muncie, Indiana 47305
(765) 281-5980

March 5, 1999

Dorothy Mae Upchurch
Director of Critical Care Services
Crichton Medical Center
4991 North Willa Way
Muncie, Indiana 47308

Dear Ms. Upchurch,

Thank you for the time spent with me during my recent interview for the position of Critical Care Educator. It was a pleasure and advantage to meet with _____ before her departure. She gave me a unique perspective on her position.

The fact that you are interested in developing an additional unit is exciting to me because I have recently been involved in a unit start-up for which I trained the new staff members. After seeing the floor plans for the new unit, I can see how important it will be within your organization.

I feel this challenging position is a good match for my background, and I am interested in pursuing it further. Again, I appreciate your hospitality and look forward to hearing from you soon.

Best regards,

Alexis Bright, RN, BSN, CCRN

SELF-EVALUATION

After each interview, evaluate how you handled yourself. Did you have difficulty handling any questions? What did you do well? What could you have handled better? Did you say anything you wish you could take back? Did they get excited about anything you said? Use what you discover to make a next interview even better.

6

THE OFFER (AND BEYOND)

You've completed the interview process, checked out the cost of living in the new area (if you're relocating), and know what the job entails. You want the job and anticipate an offer. Now you need to decide what's the lowest salary and benefit package you must have to accept this position. This is your bottom line: Anything lower and you'll turn the job down; anything higher is a plus. Then, once you accept a position, you need to think about what's beyond that — namely, leaving your old job and starting the new one.

THE OFFER AND NEGOTIATIONS

Before deciding how to respond to an offer, you must look closely at what an offer may contain. Components include:

- the hourly wage or annual salary (to get an annual salary from an hourly wage, multiply it by 2080, the number of hours you'll work per year if you work 40 hours a week)
- a signing bonus (this may be tied to a commitment to stay with an employer for a specific length of time)
- an annual bonus, based on personal or company achievements (usually offered only in management or administrative positions)
- benefits (vacation; health, dental, and optical plans; life insurance; retirement plan; tuition reimbursement; short-

and long-term disability; on-site child care or reimbursement for child care costs; and continuing education unit
reimbursement).

 ON THE MOVE   If you're relocating, the offer may also
include additional components for you to consider, such as:

- moving expenses (if offered, may cover all or part of costs
  incurred in moving)

- costs of a house-hunting trip (usually not offered for staff
  positions; some facilities may offer for other positions)

- temporary housing (rarely offered; occasionally offered for
  management and advanced practice positions). ❖

If you're not prepared, you may feel uncomfortable with
the offer stage. Because talking about salary is stressful, you
may want to tell the employer your salary requirements and
move on. But tempting as that may be, let the employer come
to you with the salary offer. Why? Because if *you* come up
with the amount, any of the following could happen:

- You may request an amount that's too high and price yourself right out of a job. Instead of getting the chance to ne-
  gotiate, you may never hear from the employer again.
  Don't forget, the salary is only part of the package.

- You may request an amount that's too low and cheat yourself out of several thousand dollars per year. The employer
  will be ecstatic when you arrive at a lower figure!

- You may come up with the exact amount the employer
  had in mind. If you do, run right out and buy a lottery
  ticket!

Remember, if *you* present a salary amount, it's *their* decision. If *they* come up with the amount, it's *your* decision.
Then, you can work from there. You may be willing to give
up a little salary for other things that are important to you,
such as location, tuition reimbursement, or child care.

What to do when you get the offer

As mentioned in chapter 5, The Interviews, if you get an offer and don't want the position — regardless of the package — inform the employer in a timely and professional manner. If you get an offer on a position that matches your blueprint and you're happy with, accept it. Ask for a letter from the employer confirming the specific points of the offer. Don't let your current employer know you're leaving until you have that letter in hand.

If it's the job you want but the salary is too low — even insultingly low — don't turn it down. Ask if you can let the employer know in a few days. Then decide what it would take for you to accept the offer. Maybe you need a higher salary, maybe a $2,000 signing bonus would do until you're up for an annual raise, or maybe you'd accept if the company would pay for you to go back to school. The more flexible and creative you can be, the better the chances for working out an acceptable agreement. In trying to be flexible, keep in mind that $1,000 a year boils down to $.48 an hour.

How you ask for more money or benefits is crucial. If you appear demanding, you send the signal that you'll be hard to work with as an employee, and the employer may not want to hire you at all. But if you use some diplomacy and flexibility, the employer is more likely to try and work with you to come up with an acceptable offer. (See *Diplomacy pays off,* page 118.)

If the employer goes back to the table and pulls strings to get you what you asked for, make sure you accept the offer. It won't speak well of you to try for still more salary or benefits at this point or to turn down the offer after you told the employer you'd take it.

If your request is reasonable (if it's in line with the salaries of other employees with similar positions and backgrounds) and the company has the money, the employer will proba-

DIPLOMACY PAYS OFF

A hiring official offers a candidate a salary of $50,000 a year to accept a challenging position. The candidate wants the position but feels the salary won't quite meet his needs. Which response do you think will help him get what he wants?

Response 1: "I'm worth at least $52,000 and I won't make a move for a penny less." (Candidates actually say things like this!)

Response 2: "I feel this position is a good fit for me, and I know I could make an immediate contribution. My wife and I sat down over the weekend to talk about it and, with her staying behind for 4 months with the kids, we just can't make the move for less than $52,000, no matter how we figure it. Is there any possibility of a $50,000 salary with a signing bonus or extra moving expenses of $2,000? That way we wouldn't take such a hit on the extra rent payments until we sell our home."

bly try and come up with a mutually satisfying agreement. But don't get too greedy once an employer is seriously interested in you. If you ask for too much, both you and the employer will lose out; you won't get the job, and the employer will have to look for new candidates.

Keep in mind that the job offer will probably be contingent upon your passing a physical (to demonstrate to the employer that you can physically do the job) and a drug screen. If you don't pass the physical, the employer may retract the offer.

LEAVING YOUR CURRENT JOB

Breaking up is hard to do—and so is quitting your job. Giving notice is never easy, no matter what history you have with your employer.

You'll probably have mixed emotions—remember how strong the emotional pull can be?—but make your departure as professional as possible. Start by typing a letter of resignation. Begin the letter with your tender of resignation, including your last date of employment. Then bring up some positive points about your time there, offer to help train your replacement (if appropriate), and wish the company success in the future. Say nothing negative (you'll only burn bridges if you do), and make a copy of the letter for your records. (See *Sample letter of resignation,* page 120.)

As a professional, you should give proper notice. Because of the responsibilities nurses have, most health care facilities require at least a month's notice. Your new employer will expect this. In turn, giving proper notice lets the employer know that you won't leave the company in a bind when you move on to another job. As mentioned in chapter 2, The Assessments, you'll probably be expected to start anywhere from 4 to 7 weeks from the time you accept the offer. Factors that affect your start date include how much notice you give, whether or not you have to relocate, and the amount of time you need off (you probably won't get a vacation for some time after starting a new job). If you have to move, you may also need a few extra days to unpack.

Once you've tendered your resignation, make every effort to make the transition as painless as possible for your current employer; help hire and orient your replacement, for instance. Give 110% through your last day. This is hard to do after you've decided to leave and are mentally gearing up for the next challenge, but you're still employed.

SAMPLE LETTER OF RESIGNATION

Leslie Joseph, RN, MSN
505 South Main Street
Owensboro, Kentucky 42301
(502) 684-5515

March 1, 1999

Eugene E. Martin, Director of Nursing
Philpot Medical Center
4455 East Vassel Avenue
Philpot, Kentucky 42303

Dear Mr. Martin,

After careful thought, I have reached a most difficult decision. I would like to tender my resignation, effective 30 days from today, April 1.

I have enjoyed being a part of Philpot Medical Center and feel my years of employment have been mutually beneficial. During my time at PMC, I have learned a great deal. However, now that I have completed my Master of Science in Nursing degree, I will be moving into a Clinical Nurse Specialist role, a position that is not available at our facility.

I will continue to wish you and Philpot Medical Center success in the future.

Sincerely,

Leslie Joseph, RN, MSN

LJ

This is also your chance to ask colleagues for letters of reference, although you may want to wait until the shock of your leaving wears off. But make sure you get those letters before your last day.

The counteroffer

You may get a curveball thrown at you shortly after you resign. Your current boss may tell you you're valuable to the organization and the company doesn't want to lose you. Then comes the offer of a raise or a promotion. Sound tempting? If it sounds too good to be true, it usually is. More than 75% of the time employees who accept counteroffers don't last 12 months—sad, but true.

So refocus. Look again at your blueprint, at why you're leaving your old job (don't forget this) and why you accepted the new one. Emotions, as you recall, are powerful. If you waiver or feel guilty because you're leaving, you'll have a rough time when your boss tells you how great you are and how much you'll be missed. If money is the only reason you're leaving, you should have asked for a raise in the first place. It's much easier and a lot less stressful than finding a new job.

STARTING YOUR NEW POSITION

Congratulations! You're about to start a new chapter in your career. You probably aren't thinking about the next career step after this—after all, you're just starting *this* job—but every day in your new position can help you prepare for that next step. Here's how to make your new job successful and help you move ahead:

- Keep a list of your accomplishments and update your résumé yearly. If you wait longer than that, you may have trouble remembering all your accomplishments.

- Set both short- and long-term goals for yourself.
- Get involved in committee work within the facility.

 ON THE MOVE   If you've relocated, get involved in your new community; it will make your overall adjustment easier. (See *Adjusting to your new life*.) ❖

- Mentor someone, and find someone to mentor you. If you're a manager, groom someone you feel has potential—perhaps someone who can cover for you when you're out and step into your position if you leave. Teach what you know, and be a resource to others.
- Get certified in your area of expertise.
- Join a professional organization.
- Be a team player.
- Be a leader.
- Be dependable.
- Be flexible.
- Give the best service you can to your customers—your patients and their families, your peers and subordinates, management, doctors, employees from other units, and anyone else you work with.
- Keep the lines of communication open.
- Address problems as they arise; don't put them off.
- Do quality work in a timely manner.
- Don't watch the clock.
- Don't gossip.
- Do more than is expected; go the extra mile.
- Work well with others; cooperate with management and coworkers.
- Present yourself professionally, both in appearance and actions.
- Keep personal problems at home (that's why they're called personal problems).
- Be able to take direction and give direction.
- Listen well.

IN REAL LIFE

ADJUSTING TO YOUR NEW LIFE

If you've relocated, you have an extra challenge: adjusting not only to a new job but also to a new life. Look at these two scenarios:

Brenda took a position in a town of 7,000 people in Iowa. She loved her job, but such a small town had the potential to be stifling. So Brenda got involved. She made the effort to make friends, took part in town activities, and even signed up for flying lessons. Three months after the move, she couldn't have been happier.

Contrast this with Lisa, who accepted a position in Los Angeles. Lisa didn't try to get involved in her community and instead focused solely on her job. Three months after moving, Lisa was miserable and lonely, even though she lived in an exciting city.

The lesson? *You* make the difference in how well your new life works. You'll get out of it what you put into it.

- Be diplomatic, not authoritarian.
- After you've been on the job a few weeks, remember your networking friends who helped you in your search. Send thank-you notes letting them know you're gainfully employed. Keep in touch with them.
- Keep learning and improving your skills. If you don't read current nursing journals, attend classes or conferences, and network with others in your area of expertise, you won't grow professionally. You'll be at the same place in 10 years as you are today. Just think how much has changed in the last 10 years!
- If you've been a job-hopper in the past, stick with this new job and make it work. Show you're committed.

Remember, what you do in your new job will be on your next résumé. You have the power to shape your career, to make wise choices that can help you successfully meet your short- and long-term goals. Keep adding to your professional network and, above all, be an *active* participant in your future!

Appendix A

STATE BOARDS OF NURSING

Before interviewing for a position, contact the State Board of Nursing in the appropriate state to find out the requirements for licensure. Some employers may require a verified license before they'll hire an applicant and give her a start date. Also keep in mind that state boards of nursing won't accept applications, transcripts, and certain other documents by fax. Contact the State Board of Nursing for more information.

Alabama

Alabama Board of Nursing
P.O. Box 303900
Montgomery, AL 36130-3900
Street Address:
RSA Plaza, Suite 250
770 Washington Avenue
Montgomery, AL 36130-3900
Phone: (334) 242-4060
Fax: (334) 242-4360
Web Site: http://webserver.dsmd.
    state.al.us/abn
E-mail: abn@abn.state.al.us

Alaska

Alaska Board of Nursing
Department of Commerce and
    Economic Development
Division of Occupational Licensing

3601 C Street, Suite 722
Anchorage, AK 99503-5986
Phone: (907) 269-8161
Fax: (907) 269-8156
Web Site: http://www.commerce.
    state.ak.us/occ/home.htm
E-mail: license@commerce.state.ak.us

Arizona

Arizona State Board of Nursing
1651 E. Morten Avenue, Suite 150
Phoenix, AZ 85020
Phone: (602) 331-8111
Fax: (602) 906-9365
Web Site: http://www.nursing.state.
    az.us
E-mail: arizona@ncsbn.org

Arkansas

Arkansas State Board of Nursing
University Tower Building, Suite 800
1123 South University Avenue
Little Rock, AR 72204-1619
Phone: (501) 686-2700
Fax: (501) 686-2714
Web Site: http://www.state.ar.us/
nurse

California

California Board of Registered
Nursing
P.O. Box 944210
Sacramento, CA 94244-2100
Street Address:
400 R Street, Suite 4030
Sacramento, CA 95814-6200
Phone: (916) 322-3350
Fax: (916) 327-4402

Colorado

Colorado Board of Nursing
1560 Broadway, Suite 670
Denver, CO 80202
Phone: (303) 894-2430
Fax: (303) 894-2821
Web Site: http://www.dora.state.co.
us/nursing

Connecticut

Connecticut Nurse Licensure
Department of Public Health
P.O. Box 340308
MS#12APP
Hartford, CT 06134-0308
Street Address:
410 Capitol Avenue
Hartford, CT 06134-0308
Phone: (860) 509-7571 (RNs)
Phone: (860) 509-7570 (APNs)
Fax: (860) 509-7286

Delaware

Delaware Board of Nursing
Cannon Building, Suite 203
P.O. Box 1401
Dover, DE 19904
Phone: (302) 739-4522
Fax: (302) 739-2711

District of Columbia

District of Columbia Board of
Nursing
614 H Street NW, Room 904
Washington, DC 20001
Phone: (202) 727-7468
Fax: (202) 727-7662

Florida

Florida Board of Nursing
4080 Woodcock Drive, Suite 202
Jacksonville, FL 32207
Phone: (904) 858-6940
Fax: (904) 858-6964

Georgia

Georgia Board of Nursing
166 Pryor Street, S.W.
Atlanta, GA 30303-3465
Phone: (404) 656-3943
Fax: (404) 657-7489
Web Site: http://www.sos.state.ga.
us/ebd

Hawaii

Hawaii Board of Nursing
DCCA Professional and Vocational
Licensing Division
P.O. Box 3469
Honolulu, HI 96801
Phone: (808) 586-3000
Fax: (808) 586-2689

Idaho

Idaho Board of Nursing
P.O. Box 83720
Boise, ID 83720-0061
Street Address:
280 North 8th Street, Suite 210
Boise, ID 83720
Phone: (208) 334-3110
Fax: (208) 334-3262
Web Site: http://www.state.id.us/ibn/
    ibnhome.htm
E-mail: lcoley@ibn.state.id.us

Illinois

Illinois Dept. of Professional
    Regulation
320 W. Washington Street, 3rd Floor
Springfield, IL 62786
Phone: (217) 782-0458
Fax: (217) 782-7645

Indiana

Indiana State Board of Nursing
Health Professions Bureau
402 W. Washington Street, Room W041
Indianapolis, IN 46204
Phone: (317) 232-2960
Fax: (317) 233-4236
Web Site: http://www.ai.org/hpb
E-mail: hprice@hpb.state.in.us

Iowa

Iowa Board of Nursing
State Capitol Complex
1223 East Court Avenue
Des Moines, IA 50319
Phone: (515) 281-3255
Fax: (515) 281-4825
Web Site: http://www.state.ia.us/
    government/nursing
E-mail: ibon@bon.state.ia.us

Kansas

Kansas State Board of Nursing
Landon State Office Building
900 S.W. Jackson, Room 551
Topeka, KS 66612-1230
Phone: (785) 296-4929
Fax: (785) 296-3929
Web Site: http://www.ink.org/public/
    ksbn

Kentucky

Kentucky Board of Nursing
312 Whittington Parkway, Suite 300
Louisville, KY 40222-5172
Phone: (502) 329-7000
Phone: (800) 305-2042
Fax: (502) 329-7011
Web Site: http://www.kbn.state.ky.us

Louisiana

Louisiana State Board of Nursing
3510 North Causeway Boulevard,
    Suite 501
Metairie, LA 70002
Phone: (504) 838-5332
Fax: (504) 838-5349
Web Site: http://www.lsbn.state.la.us
E-mail: lsbn@lsbn.state.la.us

Maine

Maine State Board of Nursing
24 Stone Street
158 State House Station
Augusta, ME 04333-0158
Phone: (207) 287-1133
Fax: (207) 287-1149

Maryland

Maryland Board of Nursing
4140 Patterson Avenue
Baltimore, MD 21215-2299
Phone: (410) 585-1900

Phone: (888) 202-9861
Fax: (410) 358-3530
Web Site: http://www.dhmh.state.md.
us/mbn

Massachusetts

Massachusetts Board of Registration
in Nursing
Leverett Saltonstall Building
100 Cambridge Street, Room 1519
Boston, MA 02202
Phone: (617) 727-9961
Fax: (617) 727-1630
Web Site: http://www.state.ma.us/
reg/boards/rn/default.htm

Michigan

Office of Health Services
Michigan Department of Consumer
and Industry Services
P.O. Box 30670
Lansing, MI 48909-8170
Street Address:
Ottawa Building
611 West Ottawa Street
Lansing, MI 48933
Phone: (517) 335-0918
Fax: (517) 373-2179

Minnesota

Minnesota Board of Nursing
2829 University Avenue SE, Suite 500
Minneapolis, MN 55414-3253
Phone: (612) 617-2270
Fax: (612) 617-2190

Mississippi

Mississippi Board of Nursing
1935 Lakeland Drive, Suite B
Jackson, MS 39216-5014
Phone: (601) 987-4188
Fax: (601) 364-2352

Missouri

Missouri State Board of Nursing
P.O. Box 656
Jefferson City, MO 65102
Street Address:
3605 Missouri Boulevard
Jefferson City, MO 65109
Phone: (573) 751-0681
Fax: (573) 751-0075
TDD: (800) 735-2966
Web Site: http://www.ecodev.state.
mo.us/pr/nursing
E-mail: nursing@mail.state.mo.us

Montana

Montana State Board of Nursing
111 North Jackson
P.O. Box 200513
Helena, MT 59620-0513
Phone: (406) 444-4279
Fax: (406) 444-7759
Web Site: http://www.com.state.mt.
us/license/pol/pol_boards/
nur_board/board_page.htm
E-mail: compol@mt.gov

Nebraska

Nebraska State Board of Nursing
Department of Health and Human
Services
Regulation and Licensure
Credentialing Division
P.O. Box 94986
Lincoln, NE 68509-4986
Street Address:
301 Centennial Mall South, 3rd Floor
Lincoln, NE 68509-4986
Phone: (402) 471-2115
Fax: (402) 471-3577
E-mail: jcampbell@doh.state.ne.us

Nevada

Nevada State Board of Nursing
P.O. Box 46886
Las Vegas, NV 89114
Street Address:
4330 S. Valley View, Suite 106
Las Vegas, NV 89103
Phone: (702) 739-1575
Phone: (888) 590-NSBN
Fax: (702) 739-0298
Web Site: http://www.state.nv.us/
    boards/nsbn/
E-mail: nsbn@govmail.state.nv.us

New Hampshire

New Hampshire Board of Nursing
P.O. Box 3898
Concord, NH 03302-3898
Street Address:
78 Regional Drive, Building B
Concord, NH 03301
Phone: (603) 271-2323
Fax: (603) 271-6605
Web Site: http://www.state.nh.us/
    nursing/nursing.htm

New Jersey

New Jersey Board of Nursing
P.O. Box 45010
Newark, NJ 07101
Street Address:
124 Halsey Street, 6th Floor
Newark, NJ 07102
Phone: (973) 504-6493
Fax: (973) 648-3481

New Mexico

New Mexico Board of Nursing
4206 Louisiana NE, Suite A
Albuquerque, NM 87109
Phone: (505) 841-8340
Fax: (505) 841-8347

New York

New York State Board of Nursing
State Education Department
Cultural Education Center, Room
    3023
Albany, NY 12230
Phone: (518) 474-3843
Fax: (518) 474-3706
Web Site: http://www.nysed.gov/
    prof/nurse.htm#addr
E-mail: nursebd@mail.nysed.gov

North Carolina

North Carolina Board of Nursing
P.O. Box 2129
Raleigh, NC 27612-2129
Street Address:
3724 National Drive, Suite 201
Raleigh, NC 27612
Phone: (919) 782-3211
Fax: (919) 781-9461
Web Site: http://www.ncbon.com

North Dakota

North Dakota Board of Nursing
919 South 7th Street, Suite 504
Bismarck, ND 58504-5881
Phone: (701) 328-9777
Fax: (701) 328-9785

Ohio

Ohio Board of Nursing
77 South High Street, 17th Floor
Columbus, OH 43266-0316
Phone: (614) 466-3947
Fax: (614) 466-0388
Web Site: http://www.state.oh.us/nur

Oklahoma

Oklahoma Board of Nursing
2915 North Classen Boulevard, Suite
    524

Oklahoma City, OK 73106
Phone: (405) 962-1800
Fax: (405) 962-1821
E-mail: oklahoma@ncsbn.org

Oregon

Oregon State Board of Nursing
800 NE Oregon Street, Suite 465
Portland, OR 97232-2162
Phone: (503) 731-4745
Fax: (503) 731-4755
Web Site: http://www.osbn.state.or.us
E-mail: oregon.bn.info@state.or.us

Pennsylvania

Pennsylvania State Board of Nursing
P.O. Box 2649
Harrisburg, PA 1710
Street Address:
124 Pine Street
Harrisburg, PA 17101
Phone: (717) 783-7142
Fax: (717) 783-0822

Rhode Island

Board of Nursing
Department of Health Professional
    Regulation
Three Capitol Hill, Room 104
Providence, RI 02908-5097
Phone: (401) 222-2827
Fax: (401) 222-1272

South Carolina

South Carolina State Board of
    Nursing
P.O. Box 12367
Columbia, SC 29211-2367
Street Address:
Kingstree Building
110 Centerview Drive, Suite 202
Columbia, SC 29211
Phone: (803) 896-4550

Fax: (803) 896-4525
Web Site: http://www.llr.state.us/
    bon.htm
E-mail: durginp@zip.llr.sc.edu

South Dakota

South Dakota Board of Nursing
4300 South Louise Avenue, Suite C1
Sioux Falls, SD 57106-3124
Phone: (605) 367-5940
Fax: (605) 367-5945

Tennessee

Tennessee State Board of Nursing
425 5th Avenue North
Cordell Hull Building, 1st Floor
Nashville, TN 37247-1010
Phone: (615) 532-5166
Fax: (615) 741-7899
Web Site: http://www.state.tn.us/
    health/

Texas

Texas Board of Nurse Examiners
P.O. Box 430
Austin, TX 78767-0430
Street Address:
333 Guadalupe, Suite 3-460
Austin, TX 78701
Phone: (512) 305-7400
Fax: (512) 305-7401
Web Site: http://www.bne.state.tx.us

Utah

Utah State Board of Nursing
Division of Occupational &
    Professional Licensing
160 East 300 South
P.O. Box 146741
Salt Lake City, UT 84114-6741
Phone: (801) 530-6628
Fax: (801) 530-6511

Vermont

Vermont State Board of Nursing
Redstone Building
109 State Street
Montpelier, VT 05609-1106
Phone: (802) 828-2396
Fax: (802) 828-2484
Web Site: http://www.vtprofessionals.
   org/nurses
E-mail: aristau@heritage.sec.state.
   vt.us

Virginia

Virginia Board of Nursing
6606 West Broad Street, 4th Floor
Richmond, VA 23230-1717
Phone: (804) 662-9909
Fax: (804) 662-9512
Web Site: http://www.dhp.state.va.
   us/nurse/regs/nursereg.htm
E-mail: nursebd@dhp.state.va.us

Washington

Washington State Board of Nursing
Department of Health Nursing
   Commission
P.O. Box 47864
Olympia, WA 98504-7864
Phone: (360) 236-4707
Fax: (360) 236-4738

West Virginia

West Virginia Board of Examiners for
   Registered Professional Nurses
101 Dee Drive
Charleston, WV 25311-1620
Phone: (304) 558-3596
Fax: (304) 558-3666
Web Site: http://www.state.wv.us/
   nurses/rn
E-mail: westvirginiarn@ncsbn.org

Wisconsin

Wisconsin Board of Nursing
P.O. Box 8935
Madison, WI 53708-8935
Street Address:
1400 East Washington Avenue
Madison, WI 53708
Phone: (608) 266-0257
Fax: (608) 267-0644

Wyoming

Wyoming State Board of Nursing
2020 Carey Avenue, Suite 110
Cheyenne, WY 82002
Phone: (307) 777-7601
Fax: (307) 777-3519

Appendix B

NURSING RESOURCES

Advanced Nursing Practice in Acute and Critical Care

Web Site: http://pobox.upenn.edu/
~jtv/button8.html

American Academy of Ambulatory Care Nursing

East Holly Avenue, Box 56
Pitman, NJ 08071-0056
Phone: (800) AMB-NURS
Phone: (609) 256-2350
Fax: (609) 589-7463
Web Site: http://www.inurse.com/
~aaacn
E-mail: aaacn@mail.ajj.com

American Academy of Child and Adolescent Psychiatry

3615 Wisconsin Avenue NW
Washington, DC 20016-3007
Phone: (202) 966-7300
Fax: (202) 966-2891
Web Site: http://www.aacap.org

American Academy of Neurology

1080 Montreal Avenue
Saint Paul, MN 55116
Phone: (651) 695-1940

Fax: (651) 695-2791
Web Site: http://www.aan.com

American Academy of Nurse Practitioners

P.O. Box 12846
Austin, TX 78711
Street Address:
Capitol Station/LBJ Building
1912 West Stassney, Suite 200
Austin, TX 78745
Phone: (512) 442-4262
Fax: (512) 442-6469
Web Site: http://www.aanp.org
E-mail: admin@aanp.org

American Academy of Pain Management

13947 Mono Way, Suite A
Sonora, CA 95370
Phone: (209) 533-9744
Fax: (209) 533-9750
Web Site: http://www.
aapainmanage.org
E-mail: aapm@aapainmanage.org

American Academy of Pediatrics

141 Northwest Point Boulevard
P.O. Box 927
Elk Grove Village, IL 60009-0927

Web Site: http://www.aap.org
E-mail: kidsdocs@aap.org

American Academy of Physical Medicine and Rehabilitation

1 IBM Plaza, Suite 2500
Chicago, IL 60611-3604
Phone: (312) 464-9700
Fax: (312) 464-0227
Web Site: http://www.aapmr.org
E-mail: info@aapmr.org

American Association for the History of Nursing

P.O. Box 175
Lanoka Harbor, NJ 08734
Phone: (609) 693-7250
Fax: (609) 693-1037
Web Site: http://www.aahn.org
E-mail: aahn@aahn.org

American Association of Colleges of Nursing

One DuPont Circle NW, Suite 530
Washington, DC 20036
Phone: (202) 463-6930
Fax: (202) 785-8320
Web Site: http://www.aacn.nche.edu

American Association of Community Health Education

7794 Grow Drive
Pensacola, FL 32514
Phone: (850) 474-8821
Fax: (850) 484-8762
E-mail: achne@puetzamc.com

American Association of Critical Care Nurses

101 Columbia
Aliso Viejo, CA 92656-1491
Phone: (949) 362-2000
Fax: (949) 362-2020

Web Site: http://www.aacn.org
E-mail: info@aacn.org

American Association of Diabetes Educators

100 W. Monroe, 4th Floor
Chicago, IL 60603-1901
Phone: (800) 338-3633
Fax: (312) 424-2427
Web Site: http://www.aadenet.org
E-mail: aade@aadenet.org

American Association of Healthcare Consultants

11208 Waples Mill Road, Suite 109
Fairfax, VA 22030-6077
Phone: (703) 691-2242
Phone: (800) 362-4674
Fax: (703) 691-2247
Web Site: http://www.aahc.net
E-mail: ConsultAHC@aol.com

American Association of Legal Nurse Consultants

4700 W. Lake Avenue
Glenview, IL 60025-1485
Phone: (847) 375-4713
Fax: (847) 375-4777
Web Site: http://www.aalnc.org
E-mail: info@aalnc.org

American Association of Managed Care Nurses, Inc.

4435 Waterfront Drive, Suite 101
P.O. Box 4975
Glen Allen, VA 23058-4975
Phone: (804) 747-9698
Fax: (804) 747-5316
Web Site: http://www.aamcn.org
E-mail: sreed@aamcn.org

American Association of Neuroscience Nurses

224 N. Des Plaines, Suite 601
Chicago, IL 60661
Phone: (312) 993-0043
Phone: (800) 477-2266
Fax: (312) 993-0362
Web Site: http://www.aann.org
E-mail: assnneuro@aol.com

American Association of Nurse Anesthetists

222 S. Prospect Avenue
Park Ridge, IL 60068-4001
Phone: (847) 692-7050
Fax: (847) 692-6968
Web Site: http://www.aana.com
E-mail: info@aana.com

American Association of Nurse Attorneys

7794 Grow Drive
Pensacola, FL 32514
Phone: (850) 484-9987
Fax: (850) 484-8762
Web Site: http://www.taana.org
E-mail: taana@puetzamc.com

American Association of Office Nurses

109 Kinderkamack Road
Montvale, NJ 07645
Phone: (201) 391-2600
Fax: (201) 573-8543
Web Site: http://www.aaon.org
E-mail: aaonmail@aaon.org

American Association of Spinal Cord Injury Nurses

75-20 Astoria Boulevard
Jackson Heights, NY 11370

Phone: (718) 803-3782
Fax: (718) 803-0414
Web Site: http://www.epva.org/
sci.html

American Chronic Pain Association

P.O. Box 850
Rocklin, CA 95677
Phone: (916) 632-0922
Fax: (916) 632-3208
Web Site: http://www.theacpa.org
E-mail: ACPA@pacbell.net

American College of Health Care Administrators

325 South Patrick Street
Alexandria, VA 22314
Phone: (703) 739-7900
Fax: (703) 739-7901
Web Site: http://www.achca.org
E-mail: info@achca.org

American College of Nurse-Midwives

818 Connecticut Avenue NW, Suite 900
Washington, DC 20006
Phone: (202) 728-9860
Fax: (202) 728-9897
Web Site: http://www.midwife.org
E-mail: info@acnm.org

American College of Nurse Practitioners

503 Capital Court NE, #300
Washington, DC 20002
Phone: (202) 546-4825
Fax: (202) 546-4797
Web Site: http://www.nurse.org/acnp
E-mail: acnp@nurse.org

*American College of
Occupational and
Environmental Medicine*

55 W. Seegers
Arlington Heights, IL 60005
Phone: (847) 228-6850
Fax: (847) 228-1856
Web Site: http://www.acoem.org
E-mail: webmaster@acoem.org

*American Correctional Health
Services Association*

P.O. Box 10
Glen Dale, MD 20769
Phone: (301) 918-1842
Phone: (877) 918-1842 (toll-free)
Fax: (301) 918-0557
E-mail: achsa@aca.org

American Diabetes Association

1660 Duke Street
Alexandria, VA 22314
Phone: (703) 549-1500
Fax: (703) 549-6995
Web Site: http://www.diabetes.org

American Geriatrics Society

770 Lexington Avenue, Suite 300
New York, NY 10021
Phone: (212) 308-1414
Fax: (212) 832-8646
Web Site: http://www.
    americangeriatrics.org
E-mail: info.amger@
    americangeriatrics.org

*American Health Care
Organization*

1201 L Street NW
Washington, DC 20005
Phone: (202) 842-4444

Fax: (202) 842-3860
Web Site: http://www.ahca.org

*American Health Information
Management Association*

919 N. Michigan Avenue, Suite 1400
Chicago, IL 60611-1683
Phone: (312) 787-2672, Ext. 254
Fax: (312) 787-5926

*American Holistic Nurses
Association*

P.O. Box 2130
Flagstaff, AZ 86003-2130
Street Address:
2733 East Lakin Drive, Suite 2
Flagstaff, AZ 86004
Phone: (800) 278-AHNA
Fax: (520) 526-2752
Web Site: http://www.ahna.org
E-mail: AHNA-Flag@flaglink.com

American Hospital Association

325 7th Street NW
Washington, DC 20004
Phone: (202) 638-1100
Phone: (800) 424-4301
Fax: (202) 626-2345
Web Site: http://www.aha.org

*American Nephrology Nurses
Association*

East Holly Avenue, Box 56
Pitman, NJ 08071-0056
Phone: (609) 256-2320
Phone: (888) 600-ANNA
Fax: (609) 589-7463
Web Site: http://anna.inurse.com
E-mail: anna@mail.ajj.com

American Neurological Association

5841 Cedar Lake Road, Suite 204
Minneapolis, MN 55416
Phone: (612) 545-6284
Fax: (612) 545-6073
Web Site: http://www.aneuroa.org

American Nurses Association

600 Maryland Avenue SW, Suite 100
  West
Washington, DC 20024
Phone: (800) 274-4ANA
Fax: (202) 651-7001
Web Site: http://www.
  nursingworld.org

American Nurses Credentialing Center

E-mail: ancc@ana.org

American Organization of Nurse Executives

1 N. Franklin Street, 34th Floor
Chicago, IL 60606
Phone: (312) 422-2800
Fax: (312) 422-4503
Web Site: http://www.aone.org

American Pain Society

4700 W. Lake Avenue
Glenview, IL 60025
Phone: (847) 375-4715
Fax: (847) 375-4777
Web Site: http://www.ampainsoc.org
E-mail: info@ampainsoc.org

American Psychiatric Nurses Association

1200 19th Street NW, Suite 300
Washington, DC 20036-2422
Phone: (202) 857-1133

Fax: (202) 223-4579
Web Site: http://www.apna.org

American Public Health Association

1015 15th Street NW, Suite 300
Washington, DC 20005-2605
Phone: (202) 789-5600
Fax: (202) 789-5661
Web Site: http://www.apha.org
E-mail: comments@apha.org

American Radiological Nurses Association

820 Jorie Boulevard
Oak Brook, IL 60523
Phone: (630) 571-2670
Fax: (630) 571-7837
Web Site:http://www.rsna.org/about/
  orgs/arna.html
E-mail: arna@rsna.org

American Rehabilitation Association

1910 Association Drive
Reston, VA 22091
Phone: (703) 648-9300
Phone: (800) 368-3513
Fax: (703) 648-0346
Web Site: http://www.iarf.org/
  AmRehab
E-mail: jim.slavin@iarf.org

American School Health Association

P.O. Box 708
Kent, OH 44240
Phone: (330) 678-1601
Fax: (330) 678-4526
Web Site: http://www.ashaweb.org
E-mail: asha@ashaweb.org

American Society of Ophthalmic Registered Nurses

P.O. Box 193030
San Francisco, CA 94119
Phone: (415) 561-8513
Fax: (415) 561-8575

American Society of Pain Management Nurses

7794 Grow Drive
Pensacola, FL 32514
Phone: (850) 473-0233
Phone: (888) 342-7766
E-mail: aspmn@puetzamc.com

American Society of Pediatric Hematology/Oncology

4700 W. Lake Avenue
Glenview, IL 60025-1485
Phone: (847) 375-4716
Fax: (847) 375-4777
Web Site: http://www.aspho.org
E-mail: aspho@aspho.org

American Society of PeriAnesthesia Nurses

6900 Grove Road
Thorofare, NJ 08086
Phone: (609) 845-5557
Fax: (609) 848-1881
Web Site: http://www.aspan.org
E-mail: aspan@slackinc.com

American Society of Plastic and Reconstructive Surgical Nurses

East Holly Avenue, Box 56
Pitman, NJ 08071
Phone: (609) 256-2340
Fax: (609) 589-7463
Web site: http://asprsn.inurse.com
E-mail: asprsn@mail.ajj.com

American Subacute Care Association

1720 Kennedy Causeway, Suite 109
North Bay Village, FL 33141
Phone: (305) 864-0396
Fax: (305) 868-0905
Web Site: http://members.aol.com/ ascamail
E-mail: ascamail@aol.com

American Trauma Society

8903 Presidential Parkway, Suite 512
Upper Marlboro, MD 20772-2656
Phone: (301) 420-4189
Phone: (800) 556-7890
Fax: (301) 420-0617
Web Site: http://www.amtrauma.org
E-mail: astrauma@aol.com

Association for Professionals in Infection Control and Epidemiology, Inc.

1275 K Street NW, Suite 1000
Washington, DC 20005-4006
Phone: (202) 789-1890
Fax: (202) 789-1899
Web Site: http://www.apic.org
E-mail: APICinfo@apic.org

Association of Child and Adolescent Psychiatric Nurses

1211 Locust Street
Philadelphia, PA 19107
Phone: (215) 545-2843
Fax: (215) 545-8107
Web Site: http://www.acapn.org
E-mail: acapn@nursecominc.com

Association of Operating Room Nurses

2170 South Parker Road, Suite 300
Denver, CO 80231

Phone: (303) 755-6300
Phone: (800) 755-2676
Web Site: http://www.aorn.org

Association of Pediatric Oncology Nurses

4700 W. Lake Avenue
Glenview, IL 60025
Phone: (847) 375-4724
Fax: (847) 375-4777
Web Site: http://www.apon.org
E-mail: apon@amctec.com

Association of Rehabilitation Nurses

4700 W. Lake Avenue
Glenview, IL 60025-1485
Phone: (800) 229-7530
Fax: (847) 375-4777
Web Site: http://www.rehabnurse.org
E-mail: info@rehabnurse.org

Association of Rheumatology Health Professionals

1800 Century Place, Suite 250
Atlanta, GA 30345
Phone: (404) 633-3777
Fax: (404) 633-1870
Web Site: http://www.rheumatology.
   org
E-mail: acr@rheumatology.org

Association of Women's Health, Obstetric and Neonatal Nurses

2000 L Street NW, Suite 740
Washington, DC 20036
Phone: (202) 261-2400
Phone: (800) 673-8499
Fax: (202) 728-0575
Web Site: http://www.awhonn.org

Case Management Society of America

8201 Cantrell Road, Suite 230
Little Rock, AR 72227
Phone: (501) 225-2229
Fax: (501) 221-9068
Web Site: http://www.cmsa.org
E-mail: cmsa@cmsa.org

Center for Rural Health Initiatives

P.O. Drawer 1708
Austin, TX 78767
Phone: (512) 479-8891
Fax: (512) 479-8898

Certification Board of Infection Control and Epidemiology

4700 W. Lake Avenue
Glenview, IL 60025-1485
Phone: (847) 375-4732
Fax: (847) 375-4777
Web Site: http://www.cbic.org
E-mail: info@cbic.org

Commission on Graduates of Foreign Nursing Schools

3600 Market Street, Suite 400
Philadelphia, PA 19104
Phone: (215) 222-8454
Fax: (215) 662-0425
Web Site: http://www.cgfns.org

Dermatology Nurses Association

East Holly Avenue, Box 56
Pitman, NJ 08071-0056
Phone: (609) 256-2330
Fax: (609) 589-7463
Web Site: http://dna.inurse.com
E-mail: dna@mail.ajj.com

Developmental Disabilities Nurses Association

1720 Willow Creek Circle, Suite 515
Eugene, OR 97402
Phone: (800) 888-6733
Fax: (541) 485-7372

Emergency Nurses Association

216 Higgins Road
Park Ridge, IL 60068-5736
Phone: (847) 698-9400
Web Site: http://www.ena.org
E-mail: enainfo@ena.org

Healthcare Information and Management Systems Society

230 E. Ohio Street, Suite 500
Chicago, IL 60611-3269
Phone: (312) 664-4467
Fax: (312) 664-6143
Web Site: http://www.himss.org
E-mail: himss@himss.org

Hospice Association of America

228 7th Street SE
Washington, DC 20003
Phone: (202) 547-7424
Fax: (202) 547-3540

Hospice Nurses Association

Medical Center E, Suite 375
211 North Whitfield Street
Pittsburgh, PA 15206-3031
Phone: (412) 361-2470
Fax: (412) 361-2425
E-mail: hnafan@pipeline.com

Institute on Healthcare for the Poor and Underserved

Meharry Medical College
1005 D.B. Todd Boulevard
Nashville, TN 37208

Phone: (800) 669-1269

International Association for the Study of Pain

909 NE 43rd Street, Suite 306
Seattle, WA 98105
Phone: (206) 547-6409
Fax: (206) 547-1703
Web Site: http://www.halcyon.com/
    iasp
E-mail: iasp@locke.hs.washington.
    edu

International Association of Holistic Health Practitioners

Bernadean University
21757 Devonshire, Suite 16
Chatsworth, CA 91311
Phone: (800) 542-3792

International Transplant Nurses Society

Foster Plaza, Building 5, Suite 300
651 Holiday Drive
Pittsburgh, PA 15220
Phone: (412) 928-3667
Fax: (412) 928-4951
Web Site: http://www.transweb.org/
    itns/index.html

Intravenous Nurses Society

10 Fawcett Street
Cambridge, MA 02138
Phone: (617) 441-3008
Fax: (617) 441-3009
Web Site: http://www.ins1.org

Joint Commission on Accreditation of Healthcare Organizations

One Renaissance Boulevard
Oakbrook Terrace, IL 60181

Phone: (630) 792-5000
Fax: (630) 792-5005
Web Site: http://www.jcaho.org

Minority Health Professions

Building 3, Executive Park Drive NE,
Suite 100
Atlanta, GA 30329
Phone: (404) 634-1993
Fax: (404) 634-1903

National Alliance of Nurse Practitioners

325 Pennsylvania Avenue SE
Washington, DC 20003
Phone: (202) 675-6350

National Association for Healthcare Quality

4700 W. Lake Avenue
Glenview, IL 60025
Phone: (800) 966-9392
Fax: (847) 375-4777
Web Site: http://www.nahq.org/amc
E-mail: info@nahq.org

National Association for Home Care

228 7th Street SE
Washington, DC 20003
Phone: (202) 547-7424
Fax: (202) 547-3540

National Association of Community Health Centers

1330 New Hampshire Avenue NW,
Suite 122
Washington, DC 20036
Phone: (202) 659-8008
Fax: (202) 659-8519
Web Site: http://www.nachc.com

National Association of Hispanic Nurses

1501 16th Street NW
Washington, DC 20006
Phone: (202) 387-2477
Fax: (202) 483-7183
Web Site: http://www.incacorp.com/
nahn
E-mail: nahn@juno.com

National Association of Neonatal Nurses

1304 Southpoint Boulevard, Suite 280
Petaluma, CA 94954-6861
Phone: (707) 762-5588
Phone: (800) 451-3795
Fax: (707) 762-0401
Web Site: http://www.nann.org
E-mail: nan84@aol.com

National Association of Nurse Practitioners in Reproductive Health

503 Capitol Court NE, Suite 300
Washington, DC 20002
Phone: (202) 543-9693

National Association of Orthopaedic Nurses

East Holly Avenue, Box 56
Pitman, NJ 08071-0056
Phone: (609) 256-2310
Fax: (609) 589-7463
Web Site: http://naon.inurse.com
E-mail: naon@mail.ajj.com

National Association of Pediatric Nurse Associates and Practitioners

1101 Kings Highway North, Suite 206
Cherry Hill, NJ 08034-1912
Phone: (609) 667-1773

Fax: (609) 667-7187
Web Site: http://www.napnap.org
E-mail: info@napnap.org

National Association of Physician Nurses

900 South Washington Street, Suite G-13
Falls Church, VA 22046
Phone: (703) 237-8616

National Association of School Nurses

P.O. Box 1300
Scarborough, ME 04070
Street Address:
163 U.S. Route 1
Scarborough, ME 04074
Phone: (207) 883-2117
Fax: (207) 883-2683
E-mail: nasn@aol.com

National Black Nurses Association

1511 K Street NW, Suite 415
Washington, DC 20005
Phone: (202) 393-6870
Fax: (202) 347-3808

National Council on Alcoholism and Drug Dependence

12 West 21st Street
New York, NY 10010
Phone: (212) 206-6770
Fax: (212) 645-1690
Web Site: http://www.ncadd.org
E-mail: national@ncadd.org

National Gerontological Nursing Association

7794 Grow Drive
Pensacola, FL 32514

Phone: (800) 723-0560
Fax: (850) 484-8762

National Institute of Nursing Research

31 Center Drive
Room 5B090, MSC 2178
Bethesda, MD 20892-2178
Phone: (301) 496-0207
Web Site: http://www.nih.gov/ninr
E-mail: info@opae.ninr.nih.gov

National League for Nursing

61 Broadway
New York, NY 10006
Phone: (212) 363-5555
Phone: (800) 669-1656
Fax: (212) 812-0390
Web Site: http://www.nln.org
E-mail: nlnweb@nln.org

National Minority Health Association

20 Erford Road
Lemoyne, PA 17043-1163
Phone: (717) 260-0409

National Multicultural Institute

3000 Connecticut Avenue NW, Suite 438
Washington, DC 20008
Phone: (202) 483-0700
Fax: (202) 483-5233
Web Site: http://www.nmci.org
E-mail: nmci@nmci.org

National Nurses Society on Addictions

4101 Lake Boone Trail, Suite 201
Raleigh, NC 27607
Phone: (919) 783-5871
Fax: (919) 787-4916

Web Site: http://www.nnsa.org
E-mail: info@nnsa.org

National Nursing Staff Development Organization

7794 Grow Drive
Pensacola, FL 32514
Phone: (850) 474-0995
Phone: (800) 489-1995
Phone: (850) 474-9124
Fax: (850) 484-8762

National Organization for Associate Degree Nursing

11250 Roger Bacon Drive, Suite 8
Reston, VA 20190
Phone: (703) 437-4377
Fax: (703) 435-4390
Web Site: http://www.noadn.org
E-mail: noadn@noadn.org

National Perinatal Association

3500 East Fletcher Avenue, Suite 209
Tampa, FL 33613-4712
Phone: (813) 971-1008
Fax: (813) 971-9306
Web Site: http://www.
    nationalperinatal.org/
E-mail: npaonline@aol.com

National Rehabilitation Association

633 South Washington Street
Alexandria, VA 22314
Phone: (703) 836-0850
Fax: (703) 836-0848
Web Site: http://www.nationalrehab.
    org
E-mail: info@nationalrehab.org

National Rural Health Association

One West Armour Boulevard, Suite 203
Kansas City, MO 64111
Phone: (816) 756-3140
Fax: (816) 756-3144
Web Site: http://www.nrharural.org
E-mail: mail@nrharural.org

National Student Nurses Association

555 West 57th Street, Suite 1327
New York, NY 10019
Phone: (212) 581-2211
Fax: (212) 581-2368
Web Site: http://www.nsna.org
E-mail: nsna@nsna.org

Oncology Nursing Society

501 Holiday Drive
Pittsburgh, PA 15220
Phone: (412) 921-7373
Fax: (412) 921-6565
Web Site: http://www.ons.org
E-mail: members@ons.org

Pediatric Critical Care Nursing

Web Site: http://PedsCCM.wustl.edu/
    NURSING/APN_info.html

Professional Resource Group, Inc.

P.O. Box 1007
Muncie, IN 47308
Phone: (800) 776-0127
Fax: (888) 776-0127
Web Site: http://www.nursequest.
    com
E-mail: jbozell@nursequest.com

Respiratory Nursing Society

7794 Grow Drive
Pensacola, Fl 32514
Phone: (850) 474-8869
Phone: (888) 330-4767
Fax: (850) 484-8762
E-mail: rns@puetzamc.com

Sigma Theta Tau International Honor Society of Nursing

550 West North Street
Indianapolis, IN 46202
Phone: (317) 634-8171
Fax: (317) 634-8188
Web Site: http://www.stti.iupui.edu/
library

Society for Vascular Nursing

7794 Grow Drive
Pensacola, FL 32514
Phone: (888) 536-4SVN
Fax: (850) 484-8762
E-mail: svn@puetzamc.com

Society of Gastroenterology Nurses and Associates, Inc.

401 N. Michigan Avenue
Chicago, IL 60611-4267
Phone: (312) 321-5165
Phone: (800) 245-7462
Fax: (312) 321-5194
Web Site: http://www.sgna.org
E-mail: sgna@sba.com

Society of Urologic Nurses and Associates

East Holly Avenue, Box 56
Pitman, NJ 08071-0056
Phone: (609) 256-2335
Fax: (609) 589-7463
E-mail: suna@mail.ajj.com

Southern Nursing Research Society

7794 Grow Drive
Pensacola, FL 32514
Phone: (850) 474-9092
Phone: (888) 509-7677
Fax: (850) 484-8762
E-mail: snrs@puetzamc.com

Transcultural Nursing Society

Madonna University
College of Nursing and Health
36600 Schoolcraft Road
Livonia, MI 48150-1173
Phone: (888) 432-5470
Web Site: http://www.nursingcenter.
com/people/nrsorgs.tcn

Visiting Nurse Association of America

11 Beacon Street, Suite 910
Boston, MA 02108
Phone: (617) 523-4042
Fax: (617) 227-4843
Web Site: http://www.vnaa.org
E-mail: vnaa@vnaa.org

Wound, Ostomy, and Continence Nurses Society

1550 South Coast Highway,
Suite #201
Laguna Beach, CA 92651
Phone: (888) 224-WOCN
Fax: (949) 376-3456
Web Site: http://www.wocn.org

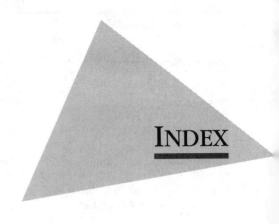

INDEX

i refers to an illustration.

i refers to an illustration.

i refers to an illustration.